I0816686

# TWO/PERCENT
# WALK WITH WEIGHT

**ALSO BY MICHAEL EASTER**

*The Comfort Crisis*
*Scarcity Brain*

TWO/PERCENT

# WALK WITH WEIGHT

## The Definitive Guide to Rucking

MICHAEL EASTER

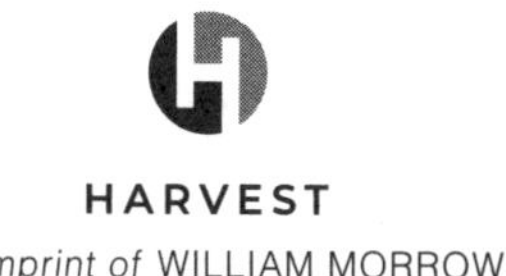

HarperCollins books may be purchased for educational, business, or sales promotional use. For information, please email the Special Markets Department at SPsales@harpercollins.com.

hc.com

FIRST EDITION

*Designed by Renata De Oliveira*

Library of Congress Cataloging-in-Publication Data has been applied for.

ISBN 978-0-06-345253-4

Printed in the United States of America

25 26 27 28 29 LBC 5 4 3 2 1

# CONTENTS

# INTRODUCTION

*Humanity did come with an instruction manual.*
*Step One: Walk.*
*Step Two: Carry something.*

In 2019, I was a 30-something-year-old professor and journalist who'd been investigating human health, wellness, and fitness for more than a decade. I'd had extended, detailed conversations with all the top minds in the fields—ranging from leading doctors to Ivy League researchers, to Nobel Prize winners, to MVP athletes and their trainers. I'd read thousands of studies, textbooks, and reports on physical and mental health, performance, mindset, and more.

I also practiced what I preached. I was a daily exerciser and health fanatic who tried all the new trends: kettlebells, CrossFit, HIIT, ultraruns, yoga—you name it.

Yet it wasn't until I was standing in the Arctic wilderness, far from civilization, that I had a realization that upended everything I thought about health and movement. Everyone I knew—even the experts—was missing the most fundamental human exercise: walking with weight.

I was in the Arctic backcountry for a month to report and research material for my bestselling book, *The Comfort Crisis.*

Over that month, I walked with weight on my back every day for most of the day.

My pack carried everything I needed to survive—clothes, food, water, shelter, sleeping bag, and so on. It became an extension of my body, and a heavy one at that—it weighed 30 to 80 pounds on any given day.

A sort of physical and mental rebirth happened to me out on the Arctic tundra.

The more I walked with weight—covering great distances across that unforgiving landscape—the more my body, mind, and spirit transformed.

My legs became like pistons—powerful and relentless.

My upper body and core became strong and bulletproof.

My endurance reached new heights—I could go all day and then go some more.

I became more durable and resistant to injuries.

Fat melted away. I began to resemble a ripped UFC fighter at weigh-in.

And my mindset expanded. I realized I was capable of achieving so much more than I initially imagined. I'd literally walked into a new realm of potential I didn't know existed.

More importantly, these changes were unlike anything I'd ever experienced during my normal fitness routines or heard of as common health advice. They were fundamentally different from what I achieved from gym workouts where I'd do 3 sets of 10 reps of typical exercises. Or from running on the treadmill or a paved road. Or by gasping my way through the latest popular high-intensity interval workout or new spin class.

Walking with weight: a physical act that was at once utilitarian, momentous, and useful in the arena of real life. There was something unique about this inherently human exercise.

After 33 days in the Arctic, I returned home and became obsessed with walking with weight. I researched its evolutionary history and all the benefits it can provide. I spoke with anthropologists at Harvard, military researchers, top physiologists, and many more thinkers about the role of walking with weight in human history, health, and performance. I uncovered scientific research going back to the 1850s and reports from Greek soldiers back before 1000 BC.

It turns out that my revelation in the Arctic was not unique. You, me, and everyone we know have all been radically changed by carrying weight, whether we know it or not.

Humans are born to carry. It is our birthright and perhaps the most important physical activity we can do. Through thousands of hours of research, I've learned that carrying weight is a missing piece of the lasting wellness puzzle. It's one of the best things we can do for our health, fitness, and mindset.

Consider this: Humans are the only species that can carry weight for long distances—and it built us into who we are. Many other animals are faster than us, stronger than us, more agile than us. They can climb better, jump higher, lift more, and beat us in a long-distance foot race. But only humans can pick up something that weighs something and haul it for miles on end.

The act of carrying weight has shaped us for thousands of years, and can help us now. I understand that sounds like a tall order, but it's true.

Over time, the act of carrying weight radically changed our bodies and minds and led us to become the apex species who ultimately conquered the globe.

Carrying allowed us to hunt and gather, build shelters and societies, and make tools. It allowed us to hold our babies close and protect them as their minds blossomed. It allowed us to take tools into the unknown so we could explore the globe and create new outposts.

But somewhere in time, we lost the consequential and critical act of carrying. It used to be an essential act for survival, but our modern, comfortable world has nearly rendered carrying moot.

We've vastly engineered carrying weight out of our lives, thanks to inventions like shopping carts, roller-bag suitcases, cars, dollies, and more. This has undoubtedly changed us, and not necessarily for the better.

Carrying weight burns more calories per mile than walking and running and melts more fat. It helps us build and maintain muscle, which allows us to age optimally. It strengthens our bones, which is critical for a resilient body and longer life. It can help prevent some of the most common maladies modern people face, like back pain and immobility. It builds endurance that can help us physically exert ourselves for days and in turn radically improve our metabolic health. It leads to a utilitarian fitness that'll help us look good, yes; but more importantly, it will make us useful and capable in the real world. The list goes on.

So how do we add carrying back into our lives in a way that benefits our body, mind, and spirit?

The simplest way is to just add some weight to a backpack or throw on a weighted vest and go for a walk. That's what I argued in *The Comfort Crisis*.

For example, the military is one group who didn't reduce carrying—they leaned into it. Soldiers have always marched with heavy loads in packs as their main form of physical training. They call it *rucking*, and it's molded them into the fittest and most capable group of humans on the planet. I wrote about the military's deep history of rucking and the benefits they've seen from it in my book.

Of course, I argued that walking with weight, or rucking, shouldn't just be limited to soldiers. It's exceedingly beneficial for everyone, especially when we use loads lighter than those warriors use.

And people listened. I began talking more about walking with weight in my *Two Percent* Substack newsletter, and my writing about the topic helped stir a bit of a craze.

I heard from hundreds of thousands of people around the world who read the book or subscribed to my newsletter and were inspired to grab a backpack, fill it with some weight in any form, and start walking.

And it changed them. These people came from all walks of life—all ages, ability levels, and backgrounds. I heard from busy moms and dads who threw on a weighted pack when they'd walk with their kids. It helped them sneak in exercise that vastly improved their health while allowing them to have more time with their family.

I heard from professional and college sports teams who began walking with weight to boost performance and maintain resilience during the rigors of the season. It increased their players' endurance while also helping them hang on to precious, performance-enhancing muscle. Some teams completely overhauled their training routines to focus more on carrying—and they went on to rack up more wins and fewer injuries.

I heard from doctors who began prescribing walking with weight to their patients. These patients ranged from age 18 to 88. Some had received scary diagnoses and needed to improve their health. Others wanted to prevent diseases from starting in the first place. Their doctors saw how safe, approachable, and powerful walking with weight could be—and their patients got healthier for it.

I heard from a Tour de France winner who found that walking with weight boosted his strength and cardio and made him more durable, helping him build a faster, stronger, more powerful body.

I heard from Fortune 500 companies whose employees began going outside on walks while wearing packs instead of meeting in a conference room. They boosted their health while building connections and dreaming up big ideas they just couldn't conjure while sitting around a table in their sterile office.

I heard from marathoners who replaced a couple of their weekly runs with weighted walking. They got stronger, found new endurance, and reduced the injuries they'd racked up pounding the pavement.

I heard from some of the country's top relationship counselors, who recommended that couples go for long walks together while wearing packs. The packs let the couples exercise together—and that extended time walking shoulder-to-shoulder allowed them to reconnect, work out issues, and remember what matters.

I heard from a group of retired women who began adding weighted packs to their morning walks. It allowed them to get more benefits from every step. Their physicians were shocked when they came back with improved health markers, denser bones, and stronger bodies that will help them outlast their peers.

Speaking of denser bones, I even heard from a NASA astronaut who returned from outer space and started walking with weight to help build back the bone density and muscle he'd lost in a zero-gravity environment.

All these people, however, had questions: Is there a best way to start? How much weight should I carry for my body size? Are there exercises that support walking with weight? What about gear? How can I do it even better and challenge myself after I've started?

Whether you're just getting started or have been walking with weight for years, in the pages that follow we'll dive into actionable strategies and tactics that will allow you to get more from every step. These practices have been tested in scientific labs and by thousands of real people.

Since writing *The Comfort Crisis*, I've gone further down the rabbit hole of walking with weight, spoken with more scientists and doctors at the most elite institutions in the world, and troubleshot hundreds of questions with real people of all ages, backgrounds, and fitness levels.

I even became part of the founding team of a company called WalkFully, which creates backpacks, vests, and hip belts that help more people walk with weight better and more safely.

*In this book, you'll learn everything you need to know about walk-*ing with weight. You'll learn why walking with weight is so important to humans and such a powerful wellness practice.

If you're new, you'll get solutions to the myriad problems you might face along the way or questions that pop into your mind. Everything from the right weight to use to the best training plans, gear, nutrition strategies, and more.

If you've been walking with weight for years or are a fitness fanatic, you'll learn new tactics to get even more benefits every time you toss on your weighted pack or vest and walk. You'll learn new skills and drills to bulletproof your body, new challenges that push your fitness and toughen your mindset, and how to optimize your walks for your goals. Any goal—

ranging from longevity to improved fitness to building a more resilient mind and body so you can walk with weight for decades to come.

The beauty is the simplicity. Simplify, simplify, simplify.

Humans are built to put one foot in front of the other, walking the earth. For all of time, we did this while carrying weight in the form of food, tools, children, and more. It gave us so much—and taught us so much about human potential. We can still get those benefits today.

Walking with weight also shifted my mindset about modern wellness trends that push us into an approach that hustles more, faster, and harder. This can produce toned muscles, but it often leaves us feeling frayed and empty on the inside, burnt out from too much intensity, and feeling like wellness is just more work.

Through the act of walking with weight outdoors, I was able to connect with deeper rhythms of life and with myself—simply by putting one foot in front of the other. I got much fitter, of course. But I also found presence over pace, consistency over intensity, and connection and intention over just another "to do" on a wellness checklist. I am more holistically healthy for it. My mind is clearer, my body is healthier, and I'm more connected to the people I love and with whom I want to be.

The changes walking with weight can bring are open and infinite. Lace your shoes, grab a pack, fill it with weight, and come with me . . .

# Part One

# WHY WALK WITH WEIGHT

# 1

# BORN TO CARRY

*Carrying is a biological norm for humans, an evolutionary conserved strategy evolved to increase survival.*

—*Bernadett Berecz, PhD*, evolutionary anthropologist

I can remember the exact moment I realized that humans are born to carry. I was in the Noatak National Preserve, in the Alaskan Arctic, on a hunting expedition. We'd struggled for weeks—but finally, after a five-hour stalk, I'd successfully hunted a caribou.

I took every part of the animal I legally could—Alaskan law says you must leave certain bones. And we'd left internal organs that humans don't eat but that would feed wolves and ravens.

The sun was an hour from dropping below the horizon. I looked out on the infinite tundra, which was ramping its way into the ground-down hills of the Baird Mountains, hundreds of miles from other humans.

I spent those wild weeks outdoors, roughing it, searching

for food in an unforgiving landscape like humans did for nearly all of time. Despite the intense nature of the landscape, however, I was more at peace than I'd ever been, feeling like I'd tapped into higher rhythms rather than the frenetic frequencies of modern life.

I hoisted my pack on my back. It weighed more than 100 pounds. Antlers burst from its top, casting a long shadow down the tundra.

I began walking. The weight of the pack pulled at me, making each step on the unstable tundra a battle. My heart rate cranked skyward. My lower body ignited, feeling pushed to the brink. My core clenched to hold my body upright.

Somewhere on that long hike back to camp—carrying this meat that would feed me and my family for months—I was struck with a great insight.

Scientists say there are 2.16 million species on earth, but only the human species became dominant and took over the globe. We explored every nook and cranny, built civilizations and cities, developed languages and commerce, and invented incredible technologies like electricity, engines, computers, and artificial intelligence.

It all started about six million years ago. That's when we stood upright and began walking on two legs. With our hands free, we started carrying things. Humans have been walking with weight ever since.

You might be familiar with the idea that humans are "born to run." That idea came from a 2004 study from researchers at Harvard University (it's also the name of a popular book based on that paper). The Harvard researchers' argument was basically this: The human body evolved the way it did so we could run long distances in the heat to hunt animals.

It worked like this: Most animals aren't efficient at cooling themselves, but humans evolved to have sweat glands and minimal body hair, we breathe in a way that cools hot air before it hits our lungs, and more. It's almost like we have a built-in air-conditioning system.

Our ancestors used their ability to keep cool on hot days to their advantage. They'd pursue animals until slowly but surely their prey toppled from heat exhaustion. Then they'd spear the animal and have food to survive.

Distance running was indeed an advantage. But during my time in the Arctic, I realized we were totally missing another, more powerful, evolutionary advantage apart from running: our ability to carry weight.

What would we do once we'd successfully run down and hunted that animal? We'd have to carry it back to camp. I was familiar with the research on how humans evolved to run long distances. But walking with weight might be our greatest and arguably most unique physical feat—yes, even more so than running. After all, many other mammals can beat us in a distance race on a cool day. None can out-carry us.

In fact, historical records suggest humans carried things *far* more often than they ran. Even as they ran down animals, they were carrying items like weapons and possibly water and food to survive the long run. Meanwhile, the other members of the tribe would be out gathering food—foraging and carrying plants all day. They'd often do this while carrying their babies, tools, and more.

When I returned from the Arctic, I visited anthropologist Daniel Lieberman in his office at Harvard. He and his colleague Dennis M. Bramble are the two researchers who discovered that humans evolved to cover great distances, often by running. He's a renowned expert who studies why the human body is built the way it is.

Lieberman confirmed that humans are "athletically pathetic" compared to many other animals, as we learned in the introduction.

But before you rage-quit all future sports and exercise because of your relative lack of athleticism, I have some good news: Our ability to cover great distances carrying items sets us apart.

As we learned earlier, our ancestors started walking on two feet about six million years ago. Back then, Earth was experiencing a global cooling period, and chimpanzees on the edge of the jungle faced shrinking fruit supplies. They were forced to travel greater distances for food. Natural selection favored the chimps who had physical traits that improved long-distance travel and height for reaching fruit. Over time, natural selection continued favoring bodies that could cover long distances—these chimps developed specialized features, like arched feet; large, angled knee joints; sideways-facing hip joints; narrow waists; and long spines that enabled long walks, while also freeing their hands to carry. They eventually became a new animal altogether: humans.

British anthropologists believe that a key reason we started walking on two legs was to free our hands to make things and carry weight longer distances.

It also changed our worldview—quite literally. We stood taller and could see higher and farther down the horizon, helping spur new ways of thinking and seeing the world.

Our free hands even kickstarted the development of our amazing brains. The anthropologist Mary Leakey notes, "From this single development, in fact, stems all modern technology. . . . This new freedom of forelimbs posed a challenge. The brain expanded to meet it. And mankind was formed."

Lieberman's 2004 "Born to Run" study published in the

journal *Nature* received a lot of attention. It led even more people to take up running, especially barefoot or while wearing shoes that mimic running barefoot, like our ancestors did.

But in the excitement around the new finding, people missed an important caveat: Humans are only superior to many other animals at endurance running when the weather is really hot. Many other animals can outrun us in a distance race in milder temperatures, where their mediocre ability to cool down isn't an issue.

Take sled dogs. When the weather is cold, they can run four-minute miles for about 100 miles consecutively and get up and do it again the next day.

But we will, in fact, kick the butt of any other mammal in a carrying competition—anytime anywhere, no matter the weather conditions. And that's exactly why we took over the world from the sweltering jungles to the frozen tundras.

When I met with Lieberman, he confirmed that our ancestors spent more time carrying than running. In fact, he told me his lab in the anthropology department at Harvard is now studying the evolution of carrying.

Lieberman pointed out that through nearly all of history, getting an item from point A to point B required that it be carried. Lieberman offered fetching water as an example. "Today we turn on a faucet and water comes out. We think that's a completely normal activity, but until fairly recently, every bit of water had to be retrieved from a well, lake, stream, or other source and carried." Sometimes these trips were short. Other times they were long—very long.

For example, in 1895, W. J. (William John) McGee, who ran the Bureau of American Ethnology at the Smithsonian Institution from 1893 to 1903, traveled to Tiburón Island in the Gulf of California. He studied the island's Seri hunter-gatherer tribe. Scientists study hunter-gatherer tribes because they provide a model of how humans lived for nearly all of human history.

In other words, they show us what life was like for roughly 2.5 million years of time. With that information, we can learn about who we've evolved to be—and the ways of living that help us thrive.

McGee stated that the Seri were "notable burden bearers." The women, for instance, would make a 15-mile round-trip excursion from the beach up into the mountains—through patches of mesquite, cactus, and agave. They'd fetch water and "rapid walk" it back to camp in big clay jugs. And when they weren't carrying water, tribe members could be seen carrying food they'd hunted or gathered, or even their children.

McGee's work provided on-the-ground evidence that humans are innately born to carry. And the academic evidence has been piling up ever since. It shows just how fundamental carrying has been to human livelihood and physicality for all of time.

Beyond watching hunter-gatherers in the wild, we have plenty of archaeological evidence showing that humans are indeed "notable burden bearers."

For example, archaeological sites show that humans were transporting heavy rocks to make tools as early as two million years ago. One site in Israel showed that prehistoric humans carried 90-pound stones short distances. But other sites show lighter boulders and stones were transported from 10 to 62 miles. Early humans had "a willingness to carry stone for hours," wrote the researchers.

Carrying gave us all sorts of bodily quirks that turned us into who we are—expanding our capabilities and imaginations.

And yet carrying as a form of physical activity has been mostly offloaded to technology. We have grocery carts, roller bags, cars, carts, and myriad other forms of transporting items—and ourselves—more easily. And we're paying the cost with our health, strength, endurance, and mindset.

So we know humans are born to carry. But it's helpful to ask: How did we make the jump from carrying in our hands to loading items in packs for our walks?

# 2

# FROM CARRYING TO WALKING WITH WEIGHT IN PACKS

On June 6, 1944, the biggest military invasion in history saved the world. It was D-Day, when Allied forces collectively launched Operation Overlord to invade Europe and free it from the Nazis.

History books and popular war films document the Higgins boats storming Utah and Omaha Beaches. For a military operation of that size to work successfully, however, groundwork had to be laid beforehand.

The evening before the boats reached the shorelines, paratroopers from the 101st Airborne Division—nicknamed the Screaming Eagles—lined themselves inside bulky, uncomfortable Douglas C-47 prop airplanes.

They took off into a dark and stormy night, flying together from southern England across the English Channel and toward the northwest coast of France. Between midnight and 2 a.m., just into France, the planes split from each other and members of the Screaming Eagles began parachuting into the black of night.

These paratrooper units landed all scattered about Normandy, and each began marching with anywhere from 50 to 100 pounds of gear: rifles, machine guns, mortars, anti-tank guns, mines, food, radios, and survival equipment.

Their mission was critical. They were to capture villages, free them from the Nazis, and help protect the surge of other Allies coming in Higgins boats. They destroyed German artillery, took over Nazi buildings and set up barracks, demolished highway bridges, and much more.

The soldiers faced a high likelihood of death during this mission, but they marched into the darkness with weight on their backs because the collective cause was greater than the individual. World War II was one of the most momentous times in history—and an Allied victory depended on the physicality of our soldiers. These men had been training for months for this operation.

When these brave soldiers of the 101st Airborne Division trained for the D-Day invasion, they didn't do so by exercising the way we often do today. They didn't bench-press or run on a treadmill in a fluorescently lit gym or spin on a stationary bike behind a screen at home. They filled a pack with heavy gear, slung it across their backs, and marched outside with other brave soldiers.

The 101st spent their time leading to D-Day at Camp Toccoa, in Georgia. The foundation of their training was excruciatingly long marches while wearing a pack weighed down with anywhere from 50 to 70 pounds.

The troops marched on uneven terrain, through dense wood, and up punishingly steep Georgia hills. This practical training translated to the battlefield, strengthened them from head to toe, exposed them to the elements of nature, and created an unwavering endurance that built true grit and an unbreakable spirit.

It also united the men. They learned that success depended on not just individual fitness but on a willingness to support each other. The shared hardship built a unified force that overwhelmed the German army. These long, weighted marches became lore of the 101st Airborne, marking them as one of the toughest military divisions to ever fight.

After the war, veterans of the 101st Division recounted that the ruck marches were transformative experiences—a key to their success on D-Day. As one military physiologist told me, "It's no coincidence that the militaries of the world have chosen walking with weight as the tool to create that physical and mental fusion of toughness."

These soldiers were part of a long military tradition of walking with weight to improve the body and mind. The military refers to walking with weight as *rucking*. As I described it in my book *The Comfort Crisis*:

> *"Ruck" is both a noun and a verb. It's a thing and an action. It's military-speak for the heavy backpack that carries all of the items a soldier needs to fight a war. And "to ruck" or "rucking" is the act of marching that ruck in war, or as a form of training for soldiers or civilians to get really, really fit.*

But because of the military's history of walking with weight and the popularity of the military term *rucking*, many people think walking with weight in a pack came from the military.

It didn't. Not even close. Rather, the military simply leaned into an act that's always helped humans find freedom, physicality, and grit.

Packs were a true game changer in human history—and they began with a clever mom, many millions of years ago.

A team of scientists from five universities worldwide studied the history of carrying and how we went from carrying with our hands to doing so using tools like packs and baskets. They explained in the journal *Infant Behavior and Development*: In all cultures across time, daily tasks must be done while caring for infants. The need to nurture infants while working likely gave rise to the use of traditional cloth and basket carrying devices.

They discovered that inventive mothers changed the course of human history:

- Two million years ago, mothers looking to carry their children more efficiently invented the first "carrying tools" by weaving together baskets and sashes.
- They put their babies inside those baskets.
- This kept the babies close and safe while freeing up the mothers' hands to gather food and do all sorts of other tasks.

Many other animals start walking almost immediately upon exiting the womb. For example, giraffes, horses, pigs, and camels are born and can quickly get up and go. Human babies, on the other hand, take 12 to 15 months to learn to walk. That's about 2.5 times longer than our closest animal relatives.

Our mothers, fathers, and community members must carry and constantly assist babies so they'll survive, which is why the development of carrying devices was so monumental.

### Why do humans take so long to walk?

The short answer is that our brains take much longer to develop. And, interestingly enough, the fact that our brains take so long to develop makes us better walkers.

One reason we're so great at walking long distances is because we have narrow pelvises, which help us walk upright and cover long distances. But these narrower pelvises have a tradeoff. They change how a baby develops while it's in its mother's womb. If a baby's brain and skull were fully formed in the womb, it would be impossible for the baby to exit at birth. A mother's pelvis just isn't wide enough.

Evolution's solution was simple. Whereas most other mammals' brains develop more in the womb, human brains develop mostly outside of it. We are basically born into the world with a brain that can only maintain some basic survival functions like breathing and eating.

But the upside is that we eventually learn to walk upright and develop the most brilliant brains in the animal kingdom. In fact, a human brain isn't fully developed until about age 25. (Take note, Mom and the Davis County, Utah, Sheriff's Office, as this partially explains this author's moronic behavior in high school.)

Once human infants begin walking, they still have a very steep learning curve. Toddlers are painfully clumsy, as any parent can attest while watching in terror as their newly walking infant explores their home and the world at large. Ancient mothers had the same worries, fretting that their infant would waltz into a sharp tree, trip and smash their head on a rock, or wander away and get snatched by a predator.

Infants also have terrible endurance. They can't walk far and must be carried for years even after they begin to walk. You might have noticed this if you've ever taken your kids to Disneyland and watched them gas out after an hour and need to be pushed in the stroller for the rest of the day.

The scientists explained that these early carrying devices "would have enhanced infant safety and mothers' efficiency while (gathering food)."

The importance of this invention cannot be understated. When these mothers created baby carriers, half of the population basically doubled their productivity. These carrying devices also protected the baby, increasing the human survival rate.

Tribes in the Amazon like the Awá, Ye'kuana, and Yanomami used tree fiber sashes to carry babies on the hip or back. Tribes in Cameroon, Tanzania, and Greenland used the skins from animals to carry infants across their backs. The Jarwa people in India used sashes wrapped around their head to carry their babies against their backs.

Of course, the invention of these early baby carriers led to an expansion of uses. Humans began using them to carry other objects to help ease daily life. They'd fill these crude packs with food, resources, and other tools to gather more food, transport more tools, and explore the unknown. Humanity exploded from there.

It was a "one small step for parents and their babies, one giant leap for humankind" moment. Many scientists think that if we hadn't invented packs to carry, we'd still be living in the Stone Age.

But as time rolled on and we progressed into modernity, we could put our kids down for longer stretches of time. We didn't have to constantly carry our children because they were now protected from danger by the four walls of our homes. Then strollers and other off-body technologies led us to carry our kids outside of our homes far less often. We also stopped carrying all sorts of other important items in packs, for example, food. We now "hunt and gather" our food inside grocery stores using shopping carts.

But there's one group of people who never put down their packs: the military.

One Green Beret told me that upon entering the military, he assumed his training would be what he'd seen in movies and on TV shows about Special Forces selection. Think boot camp instructors screaming at him to do push-ups as they sprayed water on him.

It wasn't. He was surprised to learn that rucking was the foundation of military training.

The word *rucking* comes from the word *rucksack*. German hunters first started using the term between 200 and 300 years ago to describe the waterproof backpacks they'd keep their gear in.

*Rucksack* has since then been used to describe backpacks that are designed for rougher pastimes—the type of burly, functional bags you'd keep your gear in when hunting, trekking, mountaineering, or fighting war.

By the 1920s, militaries adopted the term to describe the packs soldiers used to carry weapons and resources into war.

They eventually shortened it to *ruck* and started using the term *rucking* to describe the form of training in which they'd load their rucksacks with weight and march for fitness.

No matter what we've called it throughout time, walking with weight in a pack has always been the primary physical activity of warriors.

Assyrian king Sargon II created the first modern army in the seventh century BC. His men marched into battle dressed in armor and carrying heavy tools and weapons. Their entire kit weighed around 60 pounds.

Greek Hoplites, who were citizen-soldiers, rucked to battles with about 50 pounds of gear and armor.

Then there were the Macedonian soldiers, who historians in Australia deemed "beasts of burden." They marched to battles carrying around 80 pounds.

Obviously, going on long marches while weighed down with anywhere from 50 to 80 pounds requires a high level of fitness. If you're not fit enough to carry the load without becoming fatigued and overly burdened, you won't be fresh enough to fight.

Those Australian historians explained how Macedonian leaders prepared their fighters:

> *For the Macedonian soldier to effectively carry this load and yet still be able to function in combat, they needed to be physically conditioned. This was accomplished by vigorous battle hardening drills, which included marching [many miles] per day while carrying armour, weapons, equipment and food at a pace of [5 miles an hour]. The combined results of these changes was the creation of the fastest army the world had ever seen, with the entire army capable of covering [13 miles] a day carrying a load of between [60 and 80 pounds].*

Roman soldiers carried an average of 84 pounds to the battle site. That amount of weight is heavy no matter who you are. But it's even heavier when you consider that the average Roman soldier weighed just 145 pounds. That means the load the soldier carried was about 55 percent of his weight. For comparison, the average American man today weighs 200 pounds. That's like a modern American man walking with 110 pounds in his pack.

To prepare Roman soldiers for those heavy loads, the Roman military scholar Publius (or Flavius) Vegetius Renatus recommended that recruits be able to walk 24 miles in 5 hours with about 45 pounds in a pack.

But these early armies—and armies today—would change their loads depending on the situation. While marching to fight a far-off battle, it was necessary to carry a lot of gear and supplies for the long battle ahead. But once soldiers established a camp near the battlefield, it made sense to have them carry the lightest load possible into battle.

The less weight a soldier was burdened with, the faster he could move. As the military likes to say, "Speed is security." For example, once the fighting kicked off, Roman soldiers would ditch unnecessary gear and fight carrying 33 pounds.

Eventually, muskets replaced heavy swords and spears and war-fighting technology advanced. But the gear didn't become any lighter. For example, the British Redcoats carried about 80 pounds during the American Revolution. One reason they lost the war, historians theorized, is that American revolutionary armies carried far lighter loads, which allowed them to move faster and harder. Speed is security.

Loads crept successively higher in World Wars I and II and during the wars in Korea and Vietnam. For the wars in Iraq and Afghanistan, the average soldier was marching with about 100 pounds.

Truth be told, the military hasn't always approached walking with weight in a way that's useful for the average person.

First, the military and companies that make military-style rucking gear have put an extreme spin on walking with weight. It promotes a sort of hardcore boot camp mentality that suggests it's always best to go heavier, harder, and faster.

But that mindset neglects all the open and infinite benefits and possibilities that walking with weight can deliver. It's led people to think walking with weight is only for extreme types—but let's not forget it's something that has always been a part of human life.

And it also leads people to believe they must go hard and heavy or else they won't get a benefit. The truth is that walking with weight delivers incredible upsides even if you do it with 5 pounds at a leisurely pace.

All the research shows that making every rucking session like a boot camp can backfire. It can raise your risk of injury and suck the life out of the act.

It's not a bad thing to enjoy exercise, to make it social and fun, to take in nature along the way, and to not make it a competition. The research shows that the key to reaping the benefits of exercise is to do it consistently—and it also says we're far more likely to be consistent with exercises we actually enjoy.

Second, when I published *The Comfort Crisis*, I received various emails from veterans who told me rucking was dangerous because they'd gotten hurt doing it.

We know walking with weight is one of the safest activities you can do. But the injury risk rises as you use heavier weight or go faster—especially if you're on uneven terrain, where you can easily roll an ankle or tweak a knee.

This is why we must consider the type of walking with

weight that soldiers do. Soldiers are training to carry 100 pounds of weapons and supplies into dangerous wars. Their lives depend on their ability to do this. The "mission" is to win a war.

But that's not the mission of the average person. Most of us want to add some weight to our walks so we can get more from every step and secure an awesome range of benefits.

Exercise is a lot like medicine. Not only in the sense that it can help you avoid disease and make you healthier but also because the right dose is critical. Too little, and you won't get the benefit. Too much too soon, and it can be harmful. And that's really the case with everything:

- Eating too much food can hurt your health, but so can eating too little.
- Working too little can hurt your livelihood, but working too much can burn you out.
- Drinking too little water can lead to dehydration, but drinking too much can lead to the dangerous condition called hyponatremia.

And so it is with walking with weight. Studies show walking with weight is less risky than other acts like running.

But the risks of rucking rose as the loads the military put on the backs of its soldiers crept higher and higher. Soldiers were getting hurt, and that was impacting their ability to fight safely. This is why militaries around the world have poured millions of dollars of funding into figuring out how to walk with weight better and safer.

I've been walking with weight for more than a decade and spoken with the smartest minds in the field. We'll cover the weight you should use in part two of this book. In the meantime, here's my quick take: Find a weight that feels uncomfortable but not so burdensome that you can't go a few miles. That weight will be different for everyone. And it will change as you walk with weight more often and improve your strength and cardio.

Ease in. Start with a light weight and walk a distance you're confident you could walk without any weight. Then slowly work your way up, adding distance and weight over the weeks and months—most injuries occur when we do too much too soon.

A funny thing happened after *The Comfort Crisis* had made the rounds among veterans. Many began emailing me different messages. I heard from many vets who decided to take up rucking again—albeit with lighter weights than they used during their service.

"I hadn't put a ruck on my back since the military," one wrote. "But I'm so glad I did. I've been walking with 30 pounds every day. It's reconnected me to my past and a part of me I'd been ignoring. I've lost 20 pounds and never felt better. My doctor even asked me in my recent checkup what I've been doing, because my health numbers look great. It also really got me out of a rut I'd been in and gave me time to work up a sweat, disconnect, and contemplate while in the outdoors."

Walking with weight is indeed powerful for your health, fitness, and mindset. In the next chapter, we'll learn exactly how powerful.

# 3

# LIFESPAN AND HEALTHSPAN

After I returned from the Arctic, you'd think that I'd have been sick of walking with weight. After all, I'd spent the last month with a heavy pack attached to my body like a fifth limb.

But I wasn't. If anything, it ignited a deep interest in the act.

Walking with weight became the foundation of my exercise approach. I'd do long walks in the desert near my home with a heavy pack. I'd toss on a lighter backpack anytime I walked my dogs. And I became better for it—more physically tough, with better health, and a newfound appreciation for what my body was capable of.

After *The Comfort Crisis* came out, I heard from people all around the world who took up walking with weight—and they became better for it, too.

"I'd had two back surgeries and couldn't run anymore, so my fitness was slipping," wrote Mark, a middle-aged dad. "But I discovered I could ruck without issue, and it's been great for me physically. I'm stronger than I was when I was running, and my cardio is just as good. It's also been great for me to clear my mind."

"I started walking with weight twice a week," wrote Emma, who lives in Zurich. "I'm 52, and my core and body have never been stronger. Plus, I do it with my husband—it's the first activity we've enjoyed together, and it's brought us closer. My friends think I'm crazy, but I love it!"

"I'm a physical therapist," wrote Richard. "Rucking has really helped me to develop my core strength and balance, which so many folks lose as they age. It improved my cardio and endurance—which helps me out in almost every aspect of my life."

"Walking with weight is the key that helped me lose 50 pounds and became a 'gateway' drug to becoming healthier overall and trying other workouts," wrote Juan, a 45-year-old office worker.

"My body fat was about 25 percent and my doctor wanted me to get it to around 15," wrote Rick. "In 6 months, I added 6 pounds of muscle and dropped my fat to around 15 percent. The main difference is that I started walking with weight."

"I'm a 68-year-old woman who's always walked about 10,000 steps a day," wrote Nancy. "I started wearing a weighted pack on my walks, and it's helped me build more strength, improved my balance, and helped me keep up with my crazy dog."

"I'm a 48-year-old firefighter," wrote Jordan. "I started rucking to lose weight. It helped. I lost over 50 pounds in a year. But I got more benefits than that—my endurance was better, I rehabbed some old injuries, and I got a lot of mental health benefits from walking out in the woods, which helped with the stress of my job."

I've received more than 1,000 messages just like that. They've come from men and women around the world, from ages 18 to 88, people of all ethnic, religious, and cultural backgrounds.

Their messages add up to one conclusion: Walking with weight is a powerful form of exercise. Perhaps the most powerful. It can improve your physical health and fitness as well as your mental strength and emotional health.

It packs so much into a single exercise. It's superior to many forms of exercise because it combines weight training with cardio. You're covering ground, which works your endurance, while carrying something heavy, which works your strength.

It also gets you outside (often with other people), tests your grit, and reduces your risk of injury. It burns more fat per mile than other forms of cardio.

It's also highly practical: What's more useful and applicable to daily life than being able to pick up and carrying something? As we learned, humans are born to carry.

But we also learned that, because of its military history, walking with weight hasn't always been translated to the average person in a way that's helpful. It's turned into something of a boot camp thresher.

As one veteran named Dan wrote to me, "Being former military, I was skeptical because of how the military made us ruck," he wrote. "But I tried it with a reasonable load—and it's been a welcome return to my roots. It's a great middle ground to find strength and build some intensity at a walking pace. I'm glad I gave it another shot."

Like Dan, if we can learn to walk with weight well, we can get an incredible range of benefits that fight many of the problems modern people face. It's more important now than ever for the average person to take up walking with weight.

Chronic diseases like heart disease, diabetes, and more are rippling across the country. Mental health is at an all-time low. Function is also down, with more people unable to complete basic tasks life throws at them, like walking a long distance, carrying our kids, or lifting luggage into an overhead carry-on bin. Walking with weight is one of our best defenses against all the modern maladies that are limiting our life and ability to live it to the fullest.

In this chapter, I'll explain how walking with weight might be the ultimate exercise to enhance your lifespan—how long you live—and your healthspan—how well you live, feel, and perform in the years you have.

## IT BURNS MORE CALORIES

"How many calories do I burn walking with weight?" is a question that fills my inbox.

People message me details like their body weight, the weight in their backpack, and their pace and ask if I can give them the exact number of calories they burned, like I'm a human Apple Watch.

I get it. We want to measure a workout's impact so we know how effective it was and can make comparisons with other workouts. Not to mention, it's satisfying to see a number at the end confirming, yes, we worked our butt off.

Calories burned is an important question for both lifespan and healthspan. Burning more energy across the day vastly improves your metabolic health. Better metabolic health helps you avoid crippling diseases like type 2 diabetes, which in turn helps you live longer and better.

We often think that type 2 diabetes is caused entirely by

what you eat. But for most people, a lack of physical activity is likely more at fault. As Dr. Trevor Kashey says, “Type 2 diabetes isn’t so much a carbs problem as it is a couch problem.”

Research shows that people free from type 2 diabetes live more than 6 years longer than those who have it. What’s more, they also live better moment to moment, aren’t shackled to medications, and have better mental health and physical function, helping them enjoy life more.

Yet it’s never been easy to determine calorie burn from walking with weight. In fact, calculating calorie burn from any activity is not easy—even the number on your fitness tracker is a semi-educated but definitely wrong guess about any activity. Calculating calorie burn while walking with weight is extra challenging because:

- It’s a rather understudied form of exercise.
- It mixes strength and cardio.
- The nature of it comes with many variables that impact calorie burn: for example, the weight in your pack, the terrain you’re walking on, and how fast and far you’re walking.
- It has a muscular effect, leading you to burn more fat and build or maintain muscle. As a result, your improved body composition will likely have longer-term calorie-burning effects.

Scientists have come up with all sorts of calculations to make reasonable guesses about caloric burn, but they aren’t perfect. For example, a popular equation called the Pandolf equation, which scientists have used for years, was recently found to underestimate calorie burn.

And then, in 2024, David Looney, a mathematical physiologist who conducts research with the Department of Defense and US Army Research Institute of Environmental Medicine (USARIEM), finally gave us a great study published in the journal *Medicine & Science in Sports & Exercise* on the number of calories burned from walking with weight. So I called Looney to learn more about his work.

Marching with weight in a pack is the most important physical act of soldiers, so the military has been examining it for years.

Looney took a group of soldiers and had them walk with weight in a pack on a treadmill using different loads and at different speeds. Their packs had a weight equal to using 22, 44, or 66 percent of their body weight at paces ranging from 1 mile an hour to roughly 4.5 miles an hour.

As they walked, they had a device strapped to their mouth to measure their oxygen uptake and carbon dioxide production. By measuring the amount of oxygen the participants consumed, the scientists could determine their calorie burn.

To prove that the formula was not isolated to the one lab, Looney then "tested it out and validated it against other data that was collected in different soldiers and different populations, just to prove this wasn't a one-trick pony."

It's important to note that Looney's study included more women than previous studies. Military research has traditionally focused predominantly on men, even though more women are now entering the military. Not to mention the fact that far more civilian women are walking with weight to improve their health and fitness. What this means is that the calorie burn figures from those old studies may not apply to all people. In the study, Looney noted: "The current study represents a step in the right direction for female representation in exercise sciences."

His model is likely the best existing estimate of the calories we burn walking with weight. The graphs on pages 38–39 show how many calories you burn while walking with weight. But if you want to use a calculator to know your exact numbers, go to twopct.com/p/CalorieBurn.

To understand the graphs (or use the online calculator), you'll have to do a little math. I, too, hate math. But don't worry, we've made it easy. You'll just need to know what 10, 20, and 30 percent of your body weight is.

We're using weights equal to a percentage of your body weight instead of an absolute poundage for a good reason: If we were to give you an absolute figure in pounds, your calorie burn figure would be wrong. For example, walking with 20 pounds (an absolute poundage) would impact a 120-pound person differently than a 240-pound person. Using a load equal to a percentage of your body weight corrects for differences between the size of people and gives us a more accurate calculation.

Here's how to calculate your figures:

- For 10 percent: Take your scale weight and multiply it by 0.10. There's your poundage.
- For 20 percent: Take your scale weight and multiply it by 0.20. There's your poundage.
- For 30 percent: Take your scale weight and multiply it by 0.30. There's your poundage.

So, for example, if I weighed 170 pounds and wanted to figure out what 20 percent of my body weight is, I'd take 170 and multiply it by 0.20 to get 34 pounds.

Of course, the weight you use when you walk with weight won't be exact. For example, if you weigh 170 pounds and use a 20-pound weight, it will be about 12 percent of your body weight. But you can get "close enough" to 10, 20, and 30 percent. And if you use the online calculator, you can plug in your numbers to get your exact figures.

Each graph gives three body weights: 120, 170, and 220 pounds. That gives us a range of body sizes. You probably don't weigh exactly one of those weights, but you can make a reasonable estimation based on the position of the graph lines.

Each graph gives us three different speeds, ranging from 2 to 4 miles an hour and also shows calorie burn for 1 hour of walking with weight.

**The big takeaways:** You burn more calories the faster and heavier you ruck. "But the effective load is nonlinear," explained Looney. This means you burn increasingly more calories with more weight. That's because it's less ergonomic, or comfortable, to carry heavier weights. "More work comes from just holding that weight up against gravity versus propelling it forward," said Looney. More work = more calories burned.

But that doesn't necessarily mean you should try to load yourself down with a maximum weight when you walk. We'll cover more on finding the ideal weight and trade-offs between using lighter and heavier weights in chapter 6.

This is also why, as Looney's study showed, using backpacks burns slightly more calories than using weight vests, which are more ergonomic (we'll cover more on packs vs. vests in chapter 8).

## RUCKING ON FLAT PAVEMENT

### (ONE HOUR)

········ 120-Pound Person - - - - 170-Pound Person —— 220-Pound Person

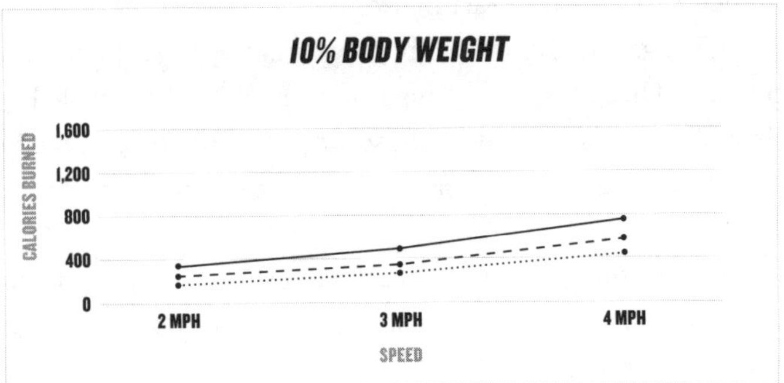


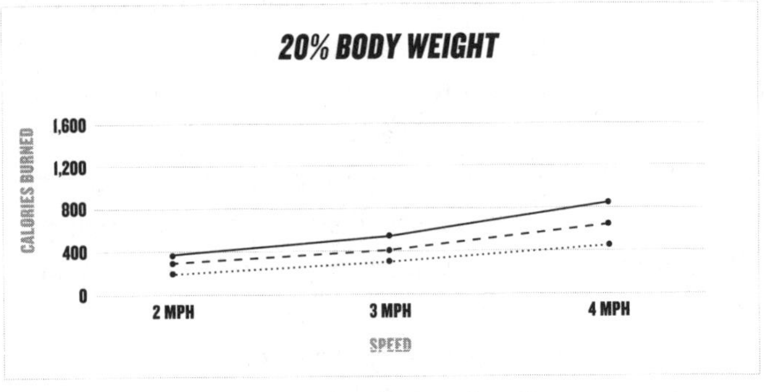


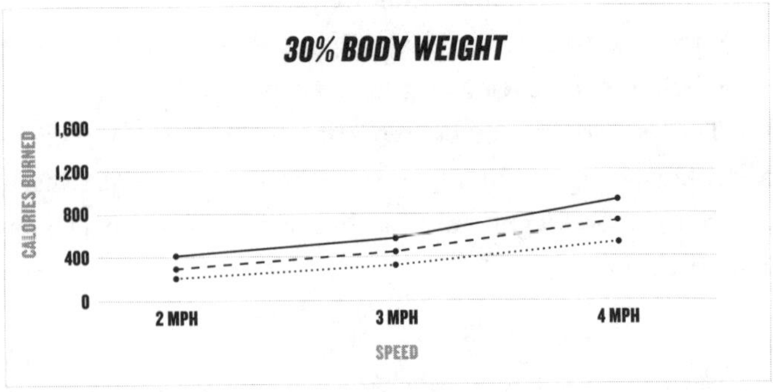

## RUCKING ON HILLY TRAIL

**(ONE HOUR)**

········ 120-Pound Person - - - - 170-Pound Person —— 220-Pound Person

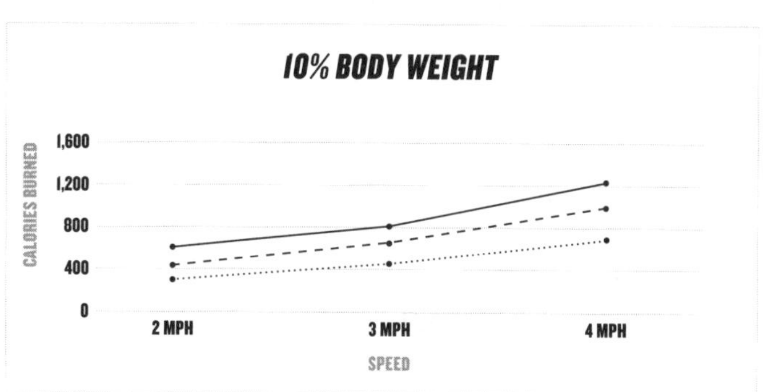


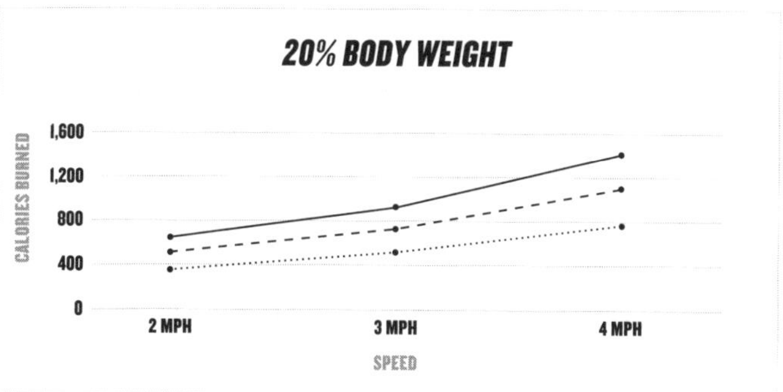


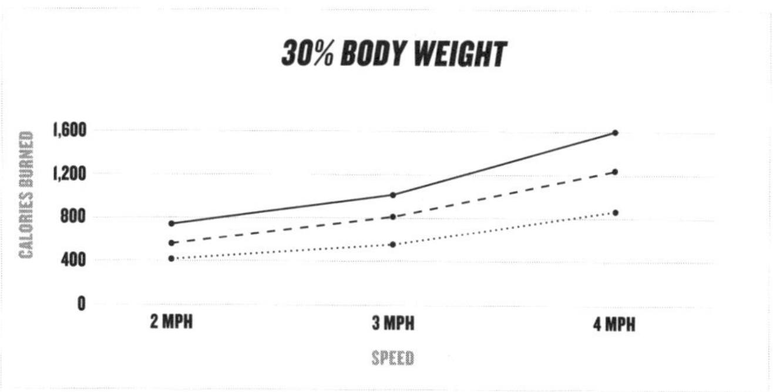

## Is my fitness watch's calorie calculator correct?

In a word: no.

Fitness trackers generally use a combination of data points to estimate your calorie burn. First, they estimate your basal metabolic rate (BMR), or the number of calories you burn doing nothing. This is why you enter your height, weight, and age when you get a new tracker. Then they combine that BMR data with data from the band's movement and heart rate sensors. Those metrics go into a formula that spits out calorie burn.

But the problem is that the calorie-burn data is always some degree of wrong. Many studies have shown that fitness trackers don't accurately measure calorie burn. Consider one study from Stanford. It compared data from fitness trackers to data from indirect calorimeters, which are basically like a gas mask you wear that accurately measures calorie burn. The scientists who performed the study wrote: "None of the [fitness tracker] devices provided estimates of energy expenditure that were within an acceptable range in any setting." The trackers overestimated calorie burn by anywhere from 27 to 93 percent.

My advice is to just ignore the calorie burn data on your fitness tracker. We usually don't have that great of a reason for tracking calories beyond just wanting a clear measurement of how "hard" we worked.

Calories give us a clear score that we can relate to

something tangible—and that "something" is usually food. For instance, burning 550 calories on a walk is like burning one Big Mac. The problem, of course, is that people often then "eat back" whatever number of calories they burned.

You can see how that is problematic if your fitness tracker overestimates how much you burn. There are much clearer ways to know how much work you did: distance, time, weight carried, and so on. For example:

- You did more work if you walked the same distance faster with the same weight.
- You did more work if you used a heavier weight but covered the same distance in the same time.
- You did more work if you walked a farther distance with the same weight.

I like tracking simple fitness performance metrics like time, weight, and distance because they're more accurate and useful than focusing on food and calories.

## YOU CAN SNEAK IT INTO YOUR LIFE AND DO IT FOREVER

We all know we should exercise. And the government's exercise recommendations are rather simple: Move your body a bit for 150 minutes a week and pick up something that weighs something (strength train) twice each week. But only 22.5 percent of Americans actually do that.

Our limiting factor isn't knowledge. Even a brisk walk counts, and we all know the basic benefits of exercise, sports, and other physical activities.

Our limiting factor is time. With that in mind, it makes sense to sneak in exercise when you can—and I'm not talking about rushing to the gym for a 20-minute CrossFit workout. I'm talking about leveling up your normal activity just a little bit, to get massive physical benefits.

Unlike running and cycling, walking with weight doesn't require special attire or equipment, and you won't have to shower immediately afterward. Unlike weightlifting, you don't need to drive to a gym, pay a monthly fee, and wait for someone to finish working out on that one machine you wanted to use.

Walking with weight is available for you to do right here, right now. Just get a pack—anything works. Fill it with an object that weighs something. Walk. It really can be that simple and easy.

Getting the mail? Toss on the weighted pack and walk down to the mailboxes. Maybe do an extra lap around the block while you're at it.

Walking your dog? Wear it.

Cleaning the house? Do it while loaded down (I did this while preparing to spend a month in the Arctic, where I had to carry a very heavy pack the entire time. It worked wonders.)

Got a work-related phone call? Don't sit. Throw on a light pack and take that call while pacing around your house or backyard or down your street.

Get creative—the only limiting factor is your imagination and how far you can stretch it. By sneaking in more activity across the day, you're beating back an early death while also enhancing your life.

Imagination not stretching? Don't worry. We're going to cover many more ways you can sneak walking with weight into your life in chapter 9.

## IT BURNS MORE FAT AND MAINTAINS (OR EVEN BUILDS) MUSCLE

When you walk with weight, you're getting those strength benefits mentioned earlier while also getting cardio. Two birds with one weighted pack, all getting you much fitter and further from death. This pairing of cardio and strength training makes walking with weight uniquely good for fat loss.

When we lose weight, we naturally lose a mix of fat and muscle. But we want to lose as much fat and hang on to as much muscle as possible.

The reason: Having a low body weight but not having enough muscle can be just as bad for you as being overweight. Research from scientist Carla Prado, PhD, shows that people with a healthy BMI but low levels of lean muscle have the highest risk of death by any cause, even compared to those with excess body fat.

Enter walking with weight. Your muscles have a strength stimulus while you're burning calories as you cover ground, which almost signals your body to "hang on" to muscle rather than burn it for fuel.

Walking with weight is better for fat loss than lifting alone because it burns anywhere from 20 to 133 percent more calories than lifting. That's simply because your body is moving effortfully the entire time you do it. When you lift, you put in effort during a 20-second set of an exercise, but then you typically rest for a couple of minutes.

It's also better for fat loss compared to running because

it actively works your muscles with weight. This stimulates muscle growth or at least tells your body to hold on to muscle. In other words, walking with weight helps you avoid the sometimes doughy, excess bulk from lifting as well as that skinny-fat look that running can sometimes produce.

Consider a fascinating study on backcountry hunters. A backcountry hunt requires walking outdoors with anywhere from 20 to 80 pounds on your back in a pack the entire time. Along the way, hunters are often eating fewer calories than they're burning because they must carry in all their food and can't pack enough; they eat little food but burn a lot of energy. (This simulates exactly what people who try to lose weight through cutting calories and exercising do: move more, eat less.)

The scientists expected these hunters to lose weight from a mix of fat and muscle. But the study results surprised them. Over 12 days, those hunters lost a lot of fat, *preserved* muscle, and saw critical fitness and health markers rise. Here are the numbers:

- Body fat: Down 14%
- Muscle mass: Up 0.1% (you'd expect a loss in muscle mass, but walking with those weighted packs prevented that)
- $VO_2$ max: Up 8.4%
- LDL cholesterol: Down 28.7%

Other research on the "gravitostat" hypothesis suggests that loading your skeletal system with a weighted vest or pack leads to more weight loss by reducing hunger. Read more about this at twopct.com/p/weight-vest-fat-loss-science.

I saw this fat-burning magic myself when I did a long

thru-hike through the American Southwest for a forthcoming book. Over 5 weeks, I lost 13 pounds but preserved my muscle mass.

And, of course, having adequate muscle mass means you can accomplish all the tasks life throws at you, whether that's participating in your favorite activity or lugging all of your family's coolers, chairs, and toys down to the beach.

## IT GETS YOU OUTSIDE

Nature is like organic Xanax. Except overdosing on it improves your mind and body rather than rendering you comatose.

As far back as 1550 BC, the Egyptians built gardens for the purpose of reducing stress. And there has been a long line of thinkers, artists, and entrepreneurs who harp on the benefits of being outside: Greek philosophers, Woolf, Thoreau, and Jobs, just to name a few.

For a while, the claims around nature being inherently good for us could have been written off as hippie, tree-hugging nonsense. But over the last few decades, scientists have proved time and time again that getting out of doors is one of the best things you can do for your mind and body.

Scientists at the University of Michigan found that spending just 20 minutes a few times a week in even the most urban nature—like a city park or tree-lined street—significantly dropped people's stress. Another study, this one conducted in Japan, found that just 15 minutes outside led to improvements in critical health markers like blood pressure, blood sugar levels, and the effectiveness of the immune system.

Some studies suggest outdoor exercise beats antidepressant medications when it comes to elevating mood and leading to lasting changes in happiness.

Yet the average person now spends 93 percent of their time indoors—and that's a major factor in our skyrocketing rates of physical and mental health issues.

This is why walking with weight outdoors can be a particularly great exercise for people with busy lives and jobs, trapped in four-walled, stifling homes and offices. It gives you time to decompress, reset, find freedom, boost your spirit, and fight against the crazies.

It can even spur creativity. Research shows walking outdoors allows your mind to bloom. One study found that people who walked for 20 minutes a day improved their concentration and ability to understand complex information.

Of course, many activities get you outside. And you should do each and every one you want. But I've found that the pace of walking with weight allows me to really take in the nature around me. To observe it, appreciate it, and feel a part of it.

And, yeah, that feels like a dose of organic Xanax. Except the side effects are stronger muscles, less fat, less anxiety, more endurance, and more happiness—the exact opposite of the 75 heinous side effects rapidly read at the end of the television ads for the real Xanax: "drowsiness, depression, headache, confusion, insomnia, dry mouth, diarrhea, nausea and vomiting, tremor, dermatitis, weight gain . . ." You get the point.

## IT BUILDS KILLER ENDURANCE

We often think intense exercise like a hard run or interval workout is the best way to improve our endurance. Going hard can be helpful, obviously.

But an emerging body of experts believes we don't have to go so hard that we feel like we're nearing cardiac implosion every workout. These scientists and doctors argue that more relaxed exercise plays a larger role in building endurance and a stronger heart and lungs.

For example, cardiologist Dr. Paddy Barrett explains that to build the most endurance, your heart needs to pump more blood per stroke. The way to do that is to make your heart's main pumping chamber larger—build a bigger reservoir for blood to fill inside.

Think of your heart being like a squirt gun. It's great if the gun shoots a powerful stream. But if the gun's reservoir is 1 ounce, you're going to get one good shot, then get your butt kicked in a squirt gun war. You want a squirt gun that has power *and* a big reservoir so you can win every battle and war.

To build a bigger reservoir for your heart to fill with blood, you must do exercise that stretches that reservoir over time. But not all exercises stretch the reservoir the same. For example, hard workouts like intervals that get your heart rate into the stratosphere make your heart better at contracting more powerfully—sort of like having a squirt gun that shoots a powerful stream—but they don't stretch the reservoir.

"Stretching" happens between 40 and 70 percent of your max heart rate—which is the heart rate zones that walking with weight put most people into. You may have heard this referred to as "zone 1" and "zone 2" exercise. In these zones, your heart rate is at a level where you're working hard but not so hard that you can't have a full conversation.

Most people will sit between 40 to 70 percent of their max heart rate by tossing on a light-ish pack or vest and going for a long walk.

This increases the challenge to your heart and lungs—but it doesn't feel like a near-death exercise experience. You can have a conversation while doing it. You can talk about things other than how hard the exercise is—and you can sustain it for far longer than exercise above this effort level.

Walking with weight will help you build a larger reservoir, and that will improve your endurance, your metabolic health, and add more years to your life and life to your years. In fact, the effects of weighted walking are about the same as those you'd get from running. One study from researchers at the US Army Center for Health Promotion & Preventive Medicine found "improvements in aerobic capacity were similar to those of [people] performing the traditional training program involving running."

I've noticed this in myself. I trail run often in the desert mountains near my home. But I've occasionally gone a couple months without running the trails. In that time, I walk with weight exclusively for cardio. And when I get back on the trails to run, I find that my endurance is just as good, if not better, than when I'm consistently running.

Of course, occasionally going fast and hard is also important. It can help your heart contract harder, making that squirt gun more powerful. And you can do that by walking faster or using a heavier weight.

Or you can do other hard and fast workouts you like, such as HIIT, CrossFit, spin classes, or anything else you can dream up. Walking with weight is one massive component of a well-rounded approach to health—but not the only part.

## IT MAKES YOU STRONGER

The US government commissions teams of our top scientists to analyze hundreds of studies to determine the ideal dose of exercise for health. In addition to getting at least 150 minutes a week of cardio, the studies also show we should perform muscle-strengthening workouts twice each week.

Recall, however, only 22.5 percent of people hit the government's rather rudimentary exercise recommendations. The biggest limiter: those two muscle-strengthening workouts, which many people skip.

The fact that 77.5 percent of Americans are missing out on strength building is alarming. Consider a study of nearly 2 million healthy people. It found that those with the strongest grips and legs were 31 and 14 percent less likely to die of any cause over a 5-year period.

Another study from researchers in Sweden discovered that the strongest people in a group were the least likely to die over 2 decades. The effect held even when the researchers removed the cardiovascular benefits of exercise.

The reason for this likely isn't that strong legs and a strong grip are magical in and of themselves. Rather, they're a marker of people who are active—a person with stronger legs likely does some cardio and weight training. A person with a stronger grip probably lifts weights or carries heavy items more often.

Another piece of research published in the *British Medical Journal* reviewed 16 different studies on the health benefits of strength. It found that people who did strength exercises like walking with weight had a "17 percent lower risk of all-cause mortality, cardiovascular disease, cancer, and diabetes."

When you walk with weight, you . . . walk with *weight*.

That weight adds a strength challenge to your entire body. Your legs must work harder, strengthening what I like to call your "go muscles": your butt, quads, hamstrings, and calves. Your upper back must hold the weight, helping it get stronger. And wearing a pack on your back works your core hard. Really hard. In fact, you can almost think of walking with weight like a moving abs workout. Core strength improves your overall health and performance and also helps protect you from injuries that cause pain to the back and knees.

Of course, if you can also lift weights, you should. That's why our weekly exercise programs in chapter 11 recommend you lift weights twice a week.

## IT'S SAFE

Years ago, one of the world's foremost physiologists, Dr. Stuart McGill, appeared on Canadian television for a debate about kids and backpacks.

Some pediatricians at the time thought kids might be doing themselves a disservice carrying heavy books in their backpacks. They didn't have evidence for this, but it seemed logical. For example, some kids might have 15 pounds of books in their pack, and sometimes those kids would even walk with the pack hanging off just one shoulder.

After the other side had laid their theories about the possible harm of walking with a backpack, McGill paused. Then he replied, "Carrying weight in a pack? That sounds like a great way to help our kids get stronger and fitter."

Then he shot down all the theories and provided actual evidence—years of research suggesting that walking with weight is arguably the safest way to boost your health, strength, and endurance no matter your age.

Research shows that walking with weight is one of the safest and most effective exercises. The best way to figure out the risk level of an exercise is to look at its injury rate over time. It's a simple calculation that indicates how many people get hurt doing a given activity over a given period.

And it's an important calculation to run: Injuries are often what hurt our health the most. When we get injured, we often stop exercising and limit our everyday movement. And when we move less every day, our most important health markers head in the direction of disease.

Maybe you've seen this in yourself or others. Perhaps you've taken up a running routine and felt great—until you hurt your knee and started moving even less than before you began running.

No physical activity is risk-free; and, of course, not being active comes with its own risks. But if we can choose highly effective exercises that have a lower risk of injury, we can avoid pain and injury and move more during our entire lifespan.

This is the key to living long and well. In other words, the secret to continuing to exercise into your nineties is to start exercising now and keep doing it. And that takes avoiding setbacks.

To understand how the injury rates of walking with weight compare to those of other popular activities like running and lifting, let's look at three studies.

## Study one

Researchers at the University of Pittsburgh tracked 451 soldiers in the 101st Airborne. Over a year, the group had 133 injuries. Twenty-eight of those injuries came from exercise. As we've learned, marching with a weighted pack—rucking—is the foundation of military training.

**The findings:** The soldiers were 6 times more likely to get injured running and about 2.3 times more likely to get injured lifting compared with marching with a weighted pack. Here's how the data broke down:

- Walking with weight: 3 injuries
- Lifting: 7 injuries
- Running: 18 injuries

## Study two

Researchers tracked the injury rates of 800 soldiers going through Special Forces assessment and selection. They found rucking had the lowest injury rate among all the fitness activities the soldiers did, with only 36 injuries. Running and the obstacle course resulted in 2 and 4 times as many injuries, respectively. Not to mention, the men were marching with 50 pounds nonstop for days on end over rugged terrain.

This is why I feel rather confident in saying that, for most of us, walking with weight is incredibly safe. Unlike those soldiers, we're doing the same activity with less weight, at a less intense pace, and for a few hours a week in our tame neighborhoods and on local trails.

## Study three

The third analysis looks at running injuries. It found that "27% to 70% of recreational and competitive distance runners sustain an overuse running injury during any 1-year period." Our inactivity in other areas of life—sitting at desks at work all day, sitting on the couch watching TV at night—seems to disturb our movement patterns and cause muscular imbalances. These often lead to injury when people start pounding the pavement.

For comparison, the injury rate of walking with weight is only slightly higher than that of walking with no weight. And walking's injury rate is roughly 1 percent. The figure climbs as a person loads a pack. But the risk is comparatively negligible at loads below 50 pounds, according to studies from the British and US militaries.

In summary: Walking with weight is incredibly safe for the average person. Load a pack with a weight that feels challenging but not soul crushing. Walk. Do it often. You'll build a robust body that lasts well into old age.

**One caveat to all this injury data:** *Military-style packs are* sometimes ill-designed for many people. The military and companies who sell military-inspired packs base the design of their packs on the anatomy of large men who need to carry more than 100 pounds.

This means their designs and materials are often inappropriate for the average person, especially women, because the packs don't suit their unique anatomy. Their design can fit awkwardly and rub your arms, chest, and other body parts raw.

That's a key reason I became a founding member of WalkFully. We're making tools for walking with weight—packs, vests, and hip belts—that suit the average person, especially women.

If you find the right pack, researchers suggest walking with weight is not only safe, it can also help you avoid injuries.

## IT CAN HELP PREVENT AND RELIEVE BACK PAIN

Back pain is popular in the sense that McDonald's is popular: over a billion people served.

- 80 percent of people experience low back pain at some point in their life.
- 25 percent of people have had back pain in the last few months.
- The low back is the most common place people experience pain and the most frequent reason people see a doctor and take a sick day at work.

- Up to a quarter of patients never fully recover from low back pain.
- People with chronic low back pain are twice as likely to suffer from depression, anxiety, psychosis, and sleep deprivation.

But when people experience back pain, they're typically offered three options: reduce your movement, take pain pills, or get surgery. These are all nearly effortless and passive—just sit, pop a pill, or lie down and get anesthetized as we cut you open—but none of them seem to help in the long run.

Reducing movement can relieve the pain, but it harms overall health. As we've discussed, a lack of activity creates all sorts of ill health effects that limit our experience of life and reduce our lifespan and healthspan.

Pills are easy. They mute pain, but they don't treat its underlying cause. They also often lead to negative side effects. Consider the opioid epidemic, which largely stemmed from people getting hooked on powerful painkillers after operations.

Then there's surgery. For one, it's expensive. For another, it often doesn't work better than exercise. One study tracked people with debilitating back pain. It found that, after 2 years, roughly 75 percent of those who had surgery were still in debilitating pain and unable to return to work. But 67 percent of those who didn't have surgery were working again.

Luckily, we have a fourth, more powerful option. Exercise seems to be the most powerful way to treat most back pain. It's not as easy as popping a pill or resting, but it's free and more effective. Side effects? Looking and feeling better, being happier, living longer, just to name a few.

Scientists recently reviewed all the existing research on what sort of exercise helps back pain. Twenty forms of exercise were included: yoga, cardio, core exercises, swimming and water workouts, Tai Chi, Pilates, stretching, and specific clinical and physical therapy methods. The good news: Doing any exercise at all was more effective than doing none.

But exercises that strengthen your core came out on top compared to traditional rehabilitation. There are many ways to strengthen your core—for example, plank exercises—but walking with weight is one of the top ways, and also delivers cardio benefits.

Carrying weight in a pack forces you to stand tall and lock down the muscles that protect your spine. Scientists in Canada found that it engages all the muscles in your core and glutes. A strong core and glutes are one of the best defenses against back pain, according to the Cleveland Clinic. This is why Stuart McGill, the aforementioned leading back health expert, often uses walking with weight to rehabilitate his patients with back pain.

## *IT STRENGTHENS YOUR BONES (WHICH IS REALLY IMPORTANT FOR NOT DYING!)*

Everyone starts losing bone density around age 30. But postmenopausal women begin losing it at a rapid and dangerous rate. This is why bone fractures are one of the biggest health threats to older women.

Aging women in the United States are 2, 5, and 8 times more likely to break a bone than they are to have a heart attack, get breast cancer, or have a stroke, respectively. But here's the thing: Osteoporosis is now becoming a growing and significant threat to men, too, according to the National Institutes of Health (NIH). And because doctors don't test men for it, they often don't realize their male patients have an issue with bone loss until those patients fall and break something.

For all of us, the decreases in our bone density are mostly due to inactivity. In the past, we performed enough daily physical labor that our bones had plenty of stimulus to keep them strong. Today, not so much. And we're paying the consequences.

A broken arm is one thing. But if you happen to fall and break a hip, you face a significantly higher risk of death. It could be a catastrophic injury. About a third of people over age 65 who break their hip will die within 6 months.

An ideal way to stop and even reverse bone loss—according to Dr. Robert Wermers, a bone disease specialist with the Mayo Clinic—is to do "aerobic walking where you're bearing weight." In other words, walk with weight.

One study had older women who were dieting wear a weighted vest and concluded, "Weighted vest use during weight loss may attenuate loss of [bone mineral density] and increase bone formation in older adults."

It's difficult to slow bone loss and build back bones no matter your activity of choice, but the research suggests that progressing the load you walk with to up to 10 to 15 percent of your body weight works well. High-impact moves like jumps also help, if you can do them safely.

So, when should you start walking with weight to protect your bones?

How about now? According to the research, the earlier in life you start walking with weight, the better you'll be. Remember that our bones start to lose density once we hit 30.

## IT'S MORE SOCIAL

A third of people say they feel lonely at least once a week, leading the US government to declare that we're facing a "loneliness epidemic." The physical and mental health effects of this epidemic are substantial.

Scientists at Brigham Young University found that it doesn't matter how old you are or how much money you have, being lonely increases your risk of dying in the next 7 years by 26 percent. Overall, they estimate it can shorten your life by 15 years. That might be why forging good relationships is a key ingredient in longevity, according to another study conducted over 80 years by researchers at Harvard.

Of course, we can do any form of exercise with other people. But walking with weight offers some social upsides that many other activities don't. Chief among them, you can have a deep conversation while doing it. The pace isn't so fast that you get out of breath.

You often don't get the same effect from running—if you're cranking out a run, you and your friends spend the time gasping for breath rather than conversing. Many sports, too, focus you so much on the sport that you can't really interact with the other person.

And it allows people to meet each other where they're at. For example, I could walk with weight with my mother, who is in her seventies. She might take 10 pounds while I'd take 30. We'd get the same fitness effect but be able to walk at the same pace together.

And walking has a long history of helping humans forge bonds. Some evidence suggests that humans have the best conversations and build the deepest connections while walking together. And it makes sense from an evolutionary perspective: For all of our history, humans have walked the Earth together side by side, often while carrying weight, for instance, food they'd foraged or heavy meat from prey after a successful hunt.

Keeping in mind all the benefits of walking together, it becomes clear why some relationship counselors are now advising couples go for long walks together. I can tell you this: The best, deepest conversations my wife and I have happen a couple miles into a long walk. I carry 30 pounds. She usually carries 10 to 20. We get more from every step with each other, connect, and hash out our future together.

Walking with weight can even help unite coworkers. A team of scientists from the University of Miami discovered that in-person walking meetings improved communication and camaraderie between coworkers when compared to sit-down office meetings.

Read chapter 9 for a guide on how to pull off walking meetings.

## IT'S REAL WELLNESS

The global wellness industry is worth about $6.3 trillion and growing. The industry, however, has left many of us feeling deeply unwell.

Consider a recent study conducted by Edelman Data & Intelligence, which found that 45 percent of people are experiencing well-being burnout—the pressure to keep up with wellness.

The report found this is largely the cause of unrealistic societal expectations, conflicting information, and feeling that we're going at it alone. We're frayed by intense workouts. We're sick of measuring our worth in the mirror or by a number on a scale or fitness tracker. We're confused by hyper-specific information on multihour podcasts about obscure, time-intensive protocols we're told we must do to be well.

I'd fallen victim to all of that. And I found the solution right at my feet: to walk mindfully and intentionally outdoors while carrying weight like humans have been for millions of years. I used my solitary walks to work out big questions about who I want to be. These walks quieted the noise so I could hear myself. I walked with others to be fully connected and committed to the people I love.

I felt supported, strengthened, and soulful—fully engaged and alive. The act became its own stance against the go-hard, grind-it-out overachiever wellness culture. And I became a better person for it.

Of course, I also got some real health benefits. The walks transformed my body in a way that decades of research suggest will improve the odds that I live long and well. Let's explore why that is next.

# 4

# BE SUPERMEDIUM

We often think our body shape and size is all about aesthetics—that is to say, looking a certain way in the mirror. And the fitness world, an industry worth more than $100 billion, is built on all sorts of aesthetic promises: get ripped, lose your gut, tone your butt, get a six-pack.

But I think body shape and size is all about *athletics*—what you can do with your body. How you use it in the world to live and function better and more intentionally every day.

You want a body type that helps you do all you want to do in life, whether it's hiking mountains, playing community sports like pickleball, chasing grandkids around, or just having fewer visits to the doctor's office.

You also want a body type that opens a world of possibilities and doesn't pin you into one lane. For example, being big and strong might be great for lifting heavy barbells in a gym, but it can impair your ability to cover ground swiftly and efficiently because you're weighed down by excess bulk. On the other hand, being light and fast can help you do well in a road race, but you'll suffer when you inevitably must lift and carry in everyday life.

Enter walking with weight. Recall that walking with weight combines cardio and strength training. You're getting both at once: melting fat and boosting your endurance while also building and maintaining strength and muscle.

Walking with weight corrects for body type:

- Have too much fat or muscle? Rucking will lean you out.
- Too skinny? You'll get stronger and put on a healthy amount of muscle.

You'll find a "just right" body type. Members of my *Two Percent* Substack newsletter and I call the type of build that walking with weight gives you "SUPERMEDIUM." It's not too thin, but it's also not too muscular. It puts you in the sweet spot. No, you may not be the absolute fastest runner or strongest person, but you'll be really good at everything and more prepared for anything life throws at you. You'll be ready for the unknown and can confidently tackle any new activity or physical challenge.

And it also turns out that having a SUPERMEDIUM body type puts you in a better position to live longer and healthier. For example, a study of more than 300,000 people discovered that those who were neither too large nor too small—a body mass index (BMI) between 22 and 23—had the lowest risk of cardiovascular disease. They also functioned better in the real world.

If you're not familiar with BMI, prepare to be. It's a measurement of your body size using your height and weight. It's an important public health measurement, and we'll reference it often in this chapter.

## WALKING WITH WEIGHT SOLVES GENDER-SPECIFIC PROBLEMS

The two-in-one corrective nature of walking with weight fixes different issues commonly faced by men and women.

Let's start with women. The data suggests many women could benefit from a little more strength and muscle. For example, only 22.5 percent of Americans meet the government's physical activity guidelines. But there's a discrepancy in that statistic: Only 19 percent of women hit the exercise recommendations, while 26 percent of men do. Why the difference? Women and men do endurance exercise at about the same rate, but women are far less likely to strength train.

Researchers in the United Kingdom found that there are a variety of reasons for this. For example, they noted that there can be a cultural stigma to women lifting weights and misconceptions about strength training, and that weight rooms are often filled with sweaty, grunting dudes who can make the scene uncomfortable for anyone and everyone.

But it's exceedingly important for women to work their muscles.

Women naturally lose as much as 8 percent of their muscle mass every decade after age 30. But when women hit menopause, hormones like estrogen decline. This accelerates age-related strength and muscle loss. This reduction can decrease your metabolism and bone density and can lead to weight gain and more fat on your frame.

Even if your weight doesn't change, having relatively more fat and less muscle sets you up for potential health risks in the long run. A study of 50,000 Canadian women, for example, found that those most at risk of death registered a "healthy" BMI but had the lowest levels of lean muscle.

And it can set off a vicious cycle: As you lose muscle, it can become more difficult to exercise. When exercise becomes harder, people often exercise less. Then they gain more fat and lose even more muscle because they're not exercising.

Other research shows that muscle acts as a massive defense mechanism if you get sick. For example, nearly 40 percent of women will develop cancer at some point in their life. But those with low muscle mass don't live as long. One theory, researcher Carla Prado, PhD, told me is that muscle improves immunity and acts as a buffer against chemotherapy drugs. Her research shows women with the most lean muscle experience 3 times fewer chemo side effects, such as fatigue, infection, and nausea—helping them power through their treatment.

By combining endurance with strength, walking with weight helps women to meet the full exercise recommendations and get stronger without setting foot in a weight room. Of course, you should also lift weights—or do body weight exercises while wearing your weighted pack or vest. That'll protect you even more. It's why we included three different 8-week training programs in part three of this book.

Now let's cover men, who often have the opposite problem. Men frequently try to build extra muscle just for the sake of it—thinking that more muscle is always better. But that isn't always the case. Piling on extra muscle for the sake of it:

1. Can take away your time participating in other health- and fitness-enhancing activities, like endurance training, degrading your overall fitness.

2. Can increase your likelihood of getting injured, which can impact your ability to exercise over the long haul (leading to a whole host of downstream problems).
3. Can lead to excess fat accumulation, which can increase your risk of health complications.

Many military recruits, for example, often find that you can't be too strong, but you can be too big. One former Green Beret told me, "The more weight you have on your body [in the form of muscle] that's not functional for the mission at hand, the more weight you have to carry around with every step. And that makes you slower and less efficient. You don't want that."

This point is backed by history. For example, movies often depict ancient Spartan warriors as bodybuilder-like physical specimens. But a military historian at the University of Oxford pointed out: "Ancient Greeks actually thought bulked-up athletes made useless warriors: sluggish, indulgent, dependent on strict diets, and unable to bear toil and deprivation."

Hence, it seems best for both men and women to have *enough* muscle. You want to be strong and muscular enough to do any job life throws at you well but not have so much bulk that it makes you . . . sluggish, indulgent, dependent on strict diets, and unable to bear toil and deprivation.

When we're strong enough, we can cover more ground outside, power up hills faster, do physical labor well, complete the physical tasks of life, and just generally live better, but we're also not weighed down by excess bulk.

There are also clear health benefits to the SUPER-MEDIUM body type—not too big, not too small. I started thinking about this after spending a week with my good friend Trevor Kashey. Saying Trevor is smart is like saying LeBron

James is good at basketball. The kid's a genius—he graduated college at 18, got a PhD in biochemistry at 22, conducted cancer research in a top lab, and now owns Trevor Kashey Nutrition, where he's helped people (many of them dire cases) lose a collective 200,000+ pounds and win Olympic gold medals.

I spoke with Trevor about muscle and body size, and he explained to me why more muscle isn't always better. He told me to think about intraspecies variation, or the differences between animals of the same species. It's a long quote, but I found that it gave me an aha moment. He said:

> *If you compare two healthy, full-grown animals of the same species, the smaller one will probably have a longer lifespan. Think of a Great Dane versus a Chihuahua—the Chihuahua lives more than twice as long on average. And there are a number of reasons for that. Like oxidative damage, inflammation, organ stress, joint stress, etc. This is why BMI is so important.*
>
> *Lots of fit but very muscle-bound men will say, "BMI is irrelevant, because it puts me in the overweight category, and look at me, I'm not overweight, I'm just super jacked!" But I take the position that huge amounts of muscle mass cause different and probably worse strain on your organs compared to an equal amount of fat. The difference between being overweight with lean mass versus overweight with fat mass is what organs get stressed out and fail first.*
>
> *Huge amounts of muscle mass means tons of vascular strain, which means more stress on your heart. Huge amounts of fat means tons of visceral fat, which leads to liver and pancreatic issues. So, let's say you have a bodybuilder and a couch potato who are*

*both in the obese category according to BMI. Both are going to die younger than necessary, but the bodybuilder will have a heart attack and the couch potato will get diabetic nephropathy . . . and probably a heart attack.*

The research suggests he's right. In the 1900s, the insurance industry noticed more death claims from their heaviest policyholders. So, a statistician at the MetLife Insurance Company found a solution. He developed a simple table using height and weight the company could use to quickly figure out the risk level of its policyholders. It worked rather well—so well that doctors began using it to guide their patients.

By the 1970s, the medical and research community fully adopted the idea. They called it the body mass index, or BMI. It's been used by the world's most influential health organizations and research institutions as a simple, quick, and free tool to assess a population's risk for weight-related diseases ever since.

To learn your exact BMI, search online for "BMI calculator."

A BMI under 18.5 puts you in the underweight category.

If your BMI is from 18.6 to 24.9, you're considered "normal" weight.

If you score from 25 to 29.9, you're considered "overweight."

Above 30 and you're considered "obese."

Anything above 40 is considered "extremely obese."

BMI has faced recent criticism because a person can have a high BMI yet be athletic. For example, you could be in the overweight category but be muscular and active. But BMI is actually very valuable if we understand its purpose and the surprising facts around it. Understanding BMI can help us make smarter health decisions.

The first thing to know is that BMI is a population health measurement. It cannot accurately tell us any one person's exact odds of any given disease (factors like genetics, exercise, leanness, and so much more alter that risk).

Instead, BMI measures how body weight impacts the disease risk for most people most of the time. But these broad strokes allow us to make rational estimations about health risks.

Imagine if a doctor wanted to get a perfect sense of her patient's health status. What would she do?

- To assess the patient's heart disease risk, she might take an echocardiogram or CT scan.
- To assess cancer risk, she might take various imaging screenings, like an MRI or more CT scans.
- To assess sleep quality, she might do a sleep apnea test.
- To assess bone health, she might do an arthritis screening.
- And on and on—test after test after test.

But doctors don't do that. Performing all those tests would be time-consuming and expensive, and the patient would wind up with massive out-of-pocket expenses. If we did that with every single checkup, our health insurance bills would be far more expensive than they already are.

In addition, unnecessary testing can do more harm than good. That's because it can lead to procedures on health abnormalities that aren't problematic and may have gone away on their own. And those procedures can lead to complications and plenty of stress. For more on that topic, visit twopct.com/p/test-downsides.

Instead, at your annual checkup, your doctor takes simpler tests. She takes your height and weight. She asks you if you smoke and if anything is bothering you. She checks your blood pressure, does some basic blood work, and maybe a couple of other things. She asks about your family history of disease and if you have any concerns. Your doctor uses your height and weight information to calculate your BMI. From there, she can quickly gauge your risk of many health issues. For example, here are some numbers:

- Up to 20 percent of cancer is attributable to having a BMI over 30. A *New England Journal of Medicine* study concluded, "The absence of excess body fatness lowers the risk of most cancers."
- A BMI of 30 or above increases your risk of type 2 diabetes by more than 200 percent.
- Having a BMI over 25 makes you anywhere from 15 to 103 percent more likely to develop heart disease. (It's the number one killer of Americans.) One study found that for each 1-point increase in BMI, heart failure risk rises 5 percent for men and 7 percent for women.
- People with a BMI greater than 30 are 680 percent more likely to develop knee arthritis compared to people who score in the "normal" BMI range. The data suggests that 69 percent of knee replacements and 27 percent of hip replacements are attributable to having a BMI of over 25. This is likely why one study found a drop in BMI of 2 or more units decreased the odds of developing knee osteoarthritis by more than 50 percent.
- Having a BMI between 25 and 30 increases your risk of early death anywhere from 7 to 20 percent. BMIs between 30 and 40 are associated with anywhere from a 45 to 90 percent increase in death by any cause. A BMI over 40, which is considered "extremely obese," is associated with

a 300 percent greater risk of death. This data is from a 14-year study. It followed 4 million adults who were disease-free at the beginning of the research period.

Problems due to a high BMI are growing globally. More than 2 billion people are now obese by BMI standards. And "between 1990 and 2017, the global deaths and (years of living in disease) attributable to high BMI have more than doubled for both females and males," found a study published in *PLOS Medicine*.

I think it's best to think of BMI in terms of gambling. For example, let's say you had a group of 100 normal-weight women and a group of 100 obese women. The research shows that the risk of heart disease for a normal-weight woman is 22 percent, while it's 39 percent for an obese woman. This means that 22 of the 100 normal-weight group would likely get heart disease while 39 of the 100 obese women would.

The important takeaways here:

- Being in a "normal" BMI doesn't mean you're risk-free. You still have a one in five chance of heart disease.
- Meanwhile, being obese doesn't automatically mean you'll get disease. You can still be healthy. It just means your risk is greater.

This suggests disease is something of a gamble, and having a high BMI seems to load the dice in favor of disease. On the other hand, having a BMI that's too low—below 18.5—is also related to various health risks.

Considering how many diseases are related to BMI . . . that's a lot of rolls with loaded dice. This is why people with higher BMIs tend to live shorter lives.

BMI is obviously less in-depth than tests like an echocardiogram, blood work, or a CT scan, but anyone can use BMI to determine their risk level. For free. In 10 seconds. No doctors or medical machines or needles involved—and, most beautifully, you won't have to haggle with the insurance company afterward. You can even determine your own treatment, too. BMI higher than you'd like? Lose weight. Too low? Gain it.

Dr. Walter Willett, the legendary epidemiologist and Harvard professor, put it this way: "Controlling weight, after not smoking, is the single most important factor for a long, healthy life."

Next is staying active—exercising in a way that works your cardiovascular system and muscles.

And that's why walking with weight is so powerful. It'll build you a body that's SUPERMEDIUM—ideally sized to resist disease and capable of whatever life throws at you.

Part Two

# HOW TO WALK WITH WEIGHT

# 5

# HOW TO START

Now that you understand why walking with weight is so powerful, it's time to actually do it. The following chapters will guide you through the ins and outs of walking with weight. You'll learn how to start if you've never tried it and how to level up once you're hooked (and you will be).

You'll learn answers to many of the most common questions, like how much weight you should use, the difference between walking with a weighted backpack versus vest, and much more. I'll also provide warm-up exercises, training plans, and gear hacks that will help you push your limits and expand your ability to walk with weight—improving your body and mind.

You can never be too good at the basics. So, while this particular chapter is geared toward a person who's new to walking with weight, those accustomed to walking with weight will also gain important insights. As my friend and thriller writer Jack Carr wrote, "Being an 'expert' in anything means doing the basics exceptionally well."

You'll learn:

- The pack you should start with.
- The types of weights you can use to load the pack.
- The amount of weight you should start with.
- How to load the pack.
- How to adjust the straps.
- The type of shoes you should wear.
- The pace at which you should start walking.
- What your posture should look like as you walk with weight.
- How often and far you should walk at first.

Many readers of my Substack newsletter, *Two Percent*, have told me that what got them started was not overthinking things. They simply used gear they had on hand and started walking.

One reader, a tech worker named Bryan, said, "I kept it simple. I threw on some shoes and a backpack with some books in it and got out the door. I walked in my neighborhood, with no car to reach a starting point or special destination in mind. That ease of entry worked. Now, I think of walking with weight as my MVP (minimum viable product). I do it when I'm pressed for time or have breaks in my workday."

Another reader, Caroline, gave this advice to people new to walking with weight: "I tend to overthink most things, but I pressed back against that. I grabbed a pack, filled it with some weight, and started walking. That really helped me avoid paralysis by analysis. Once I started, I loved it and have kept doing it."

As the poet William Wordsworth wrote, "To begin, begin."

## GRAB A BACKPACK

When you decide you want to walk with weight, it's tempting to go out and buy all kinds of new gear: a pack or vest specifically designed for walking with weight and special weights that fit snugly into the pack.

I think this gear can be great for the dedicated walker because it makes your experience more comfortable and streamlined, but I'd caution against spending a lot of money on new gear when you start.

Maybe you've experienced this before: You got excited about a new fitness activity and went out and purchased a bunch of equipment. Perhaps it was a Peloton bike for $2,000 or a kettlebell for $200. You used the equipment often for the first week. Then you used it a few times the second week. You used it once or twice the third and fourth week—and then, eventually, the Peloton became a clothes rack and the kettlebell became an expensive doorstop.

I'll admit that buying a bunch of cool new gear can incentivize *some* people to dive headfirst into a new activity. So, if you're the person who bought the Peloton or kettlebell and used them religiously, then perhaps you'd benefit from buying special gear (we'll cover gear options in chapter 8).

Yet for most people most of the time, it makes sense to use what you have at home first. Walking with weight is indeed a wonderful and truly egalitarian activity because you already have what you need to begin: a backpack and something that weighs something. The backpack you use at first might be some old bookbag you had in college, a pack you bought as a carry-on for travel, or a hiking backpack you got from an outdoor store. It doesn't matter.

Grab a pack. Load it. Go for a walk. To begin, begin—it really can be that simple.

Using what you already have allows you to get used to walking with weight and develop the habit. It can also help you determine what you do and don't like about gear before you spend any money. And it eliminates your excuses. How many of us avoid exercise because we think we don't have the right tools for the job? As *Two Percent* reader Monique put it, "I like to use an old beat-up pack. . . . It kind of makes it feel tougher and more badass."

You may find you never need to upgrade to special equipment. I know plenty of people who have been walking with weight for years with an old hiking backpack they used for their first walk, like Monique.

## FIND SOME WEIGHTS

You can purchase weights designed specifically for walking with weight—think rucking-specific packs and vests. The weights often fit into the laptop sleeve of a pack. Like with packs, however, I recommend you start with whatever you have lying around the house. Find something that weighs something and put it in your pack.

Of course, some things are better to use as weights than other things. Here are a few go-to options you probably already have at home or can buy for less than $30. Consider wrapping loose weights—like bottles, sand, bricks, dumbbells, and books—in a towel. The towel secures and pads the weights so they don't jostle around and dig into your back.

- **A bag of rice or sand**
  You could grab some sand from the backyard and double bag it in a lawn and leaf bag. You can also buy bags of playground sand from a hardware store. The bags are usually sold at 50 pounds, so just pour some out. Another option is a bag of rice from the grocery store.

With the options above, double bag it or tape it so it doesn't burst.

- **A hydration bladder, bottles, and/or water jugs**
  The nice thing about using water as a weight is that, if you have too much weight, you can always pour some water out. This can be especially helpful when you start.
- **Bricks**
  One brick weighs 4.5 pounds. Wrap two, three, or four bricks in duct tape as a flat unit. Wrap the bricks in a towel for comfort.
- **Books**
  Load them up, just like you did in grade school.
- **Dumbbells**
  "I use a few 5-pound dumbbells in my pack," wrote *Two Percent* reader Diane. Prop them vertically in the bag, wrapped in a towel or T-shirt.
- **Regular outdoor gear**
  One reader, Joyce, wrote to me, "I walk with my regular hiking stuff in my hiking pack. It's about 20 pounds." For example, a gallon of water, a jet boil stove, a tent, and more. This is a particularly good option for people who are using walking with weight to train for an upcoming outdoor adventure. It'll get you used to your gear, loading it, and having it on your back.
- **Weight plates**
  Yes, you'll have to spend a bit of money. But you can get a steel plate or sand plate that fits into a laptop sleeve starting at $30 on Amazon.

If you're wondering if you should use a weight vest, read chapter 8. It breaks down the differences between walking with a weighted pack versus a vest. If you don't already own a weight vest and are considering buying one, hold off until you read the chapter—some vests are far better than others.

## HOW MUCH WEIGHT TO START WITH

Walking with weight is beautiful in its simplicity. There are only a few ways you can screw it up. Using an inappropriate weight is the most frequent mistake people make when they start.

But men and women often have opposite problems.

Men try to be heroes. They usually go too heavy, too soon. This can result in a miserable first-time experience, like playing your first round of golf on an extremely hard course or skiing a black diamond on your first run ever. The act will be no fun, your shoulders will be sore because they aren't ready, and it can result in overuse issues, especially if you use too much weight frequently. Decades of military data show that frequently walking with very heavy loads raises the risk of overuse injuries.

Women, on the other hand, often go too light. It makes their initial walks more enjoyable—which is great because it helps develop the habit—but leaves some benefits off the table. Using weight that is too light can hold you back from getting a more powerful workout stimulus.

So, there's an inherent tension to the question of how much weight we should use: We need to load our pack heavy enough to get a great workout stimulus but not so heavy that we overdo it and suck all the fun out of the act. As a general rule, most active men can start with 15 to 35 pounds. Active women usually do great starting with 10 to 20 pounds. These weights should feel challenging but not soul-crushing.

As you walk, you definitely want to "feel" the weight on your body. Your core and shoulders should feel engaged. On hills, your legs will feel like they're working harder. Your heart rate should be higher than it is on a normal walk. But the walk shouldn't feel like a death march.

If you want to get more specific, try starting with anywhere from 10 to 15 percent of your body weight. That means if you weigh 150 pounds, you'd use anywhere from 15 to 22.5 pounds. But use your best judgment. If 10 percent of your body weight feels too heavy at first, go lighter. Soon enough, that 10 percent will feel easy.

Once you've done a few walks with a comfortable but challenging weight, feel free to add more weight. But be aware that walking with weight somehow breaks the laws of physics. As my friend and founder of Whole30, Melissa Urban, said when she increased the weight she used from 20 to 30 pounds: "Thirty pounds somehow feels like it weighs five times more than twenty pounds."

In cases like that, even though we've added only 10 pounds—which doesn't seem like much—10 pounds makes the pack 50 percent heavier, which is actually quite a bump. Think of it like increasing your speed as a runner: If you ran a mile 50 percent faster, it's a significant fitness push.

Of course, if your starting weight feels far too easy, add more weight. I've had friends like podcaster Dr. Peter Attia who started at 30 pounds and immediately bumped up to 45.

As you become stronger, you can push the envelope (we'll cover the heaviest weight you should use in the next chapter).

If you're wondering how much your pack weighs once you load it with weight, do the following:

- Step on a scale. Write down your weight.
- Now put your loaded pack on and step on the scale again. Write down your weight.

- Calculate the difference between the two numbers.
- For example, let's say I weighed myself and found I weigh 170 pounds. If I placed the weight on my back and found I weighed 205, my pack would weigh 35 pounds.

## HOW TO LOAD THE PACK

In general, it's best to have the weight closer to your back and secure in the pack. For example, it shouldn't be leaning outward or sideways in the bag nor should it be flopping around.

A few problems can arise when your weight is loaded incorrectly. A study published in the journal *Military Medicine* and led by army health researchers concluded, "Locating the load center of mass as close as possible to the body center of mass results in the lowest energy cost and tends to keep the body in an upright position similar to unloaded walking." In other words, the farther away the weight is from your back, the more you'll have to fight the weight—and that can alter your stride and posture in ways that make you less efficient.

Those same army researchers also looked at how high in the pack the weight should be. For example, should it be at the very bottom of the bag, or should you try to elevate it so it's closer to the top of the bag? This might seem like a pedantic question. As we learned, walking with weight is quite safe, and the injury risks are low. But if we can easily minimize risks by loading the pack one way instead of another, we may as well take the smarter option.

They found that for even terrain, like walking on a road, sidewalk, or well-groomed trail, keeping the weight higher in the bag is ideal. That's because, when the load is lower in the pack, you must lean farther forward to walk with the weight balanced over your feet. They wrote that having your body leaning farther over your feet can increase the likelihood that you'll strain your feet.

So, for most walks, having the weight higher is better. That said, the researchers found that it might make sense to keep the load lower in the pack on uneven terrain simply because your likelihood of unexpectedly stumbling is higher on uneven terrain, and when the weight is higher in the pack, it's harder to recover from a stumble.

In short, most of the time you'll want the weight next to your back and higher in the pack; if you're on a really rocky and uneven trail, having the weight lower might be better.

An easy way to elevate the weight in your pack is to place a yoga block, a few folded-up towels, or a small cardboard box at the bottom of your pack and set whatever weight you're using on top of that platform. Wrapping your weights in something like a towel will keep them together as you elevate them.

## WHAT SHOES TO WEAR

Soldiers are known to wear burly, overbuilt boots, which has led many people to assume they should also use big boots when walking with weight. But big boots come with downsides for the average person.

Military researchers found that the more supportive and overbuilt a shoe—think big, heavy combat boots—the more energy it takes to walk in them. For example, when the researchers compared the differences between walking in burly military boots and standard running shoes, they found that walking in boots took 6 to 9 percent more energy.

The military has extensively studied footwear because

shoes directly affect injury risk. One military study is particularly informative for the average person because it compared the effects of walking with weight in standard, supportive running shoes to walking in minimalist shoes, which are shoes that offer little support and mimic how we walk barefoot. These two categories of shoes are what you'd find at the average sporting goods or outdoor store.

Military and university researchers recruited about 1,000 cadets. The cadets entered a 9-week basic training course at the same age and fitness level. The researchers had half of the participants wear standard, supportive running shoes and the other half wear minimalist shoes.

When the 9 weeks were up, roughly 18 percent of the soldiers had sustained a lower body injury. But the ones in the minimalist shoes comprised most of those injured.

The scientists wrote that the soldiers wearing more supportive shoes were "49% less likely to incur any type of lower extremity injury and 52% less likely to incur an overuse lower extremity injury than cadets wearing [minimalist shoes]."

When walking with weight, we need to stabilize that load, and our only connection to the ground is through our feet. More supportive shoes reduce the stabilization work our feet and lower body must perform, especially as we walk faster or carry more weight.

The bottom line: Choose a comfortable running or walking shoe with moderate support. Heavy boots waste energy, while minimalist shoes increase injury risk. Most people do well with shoes offering some arch support, cushioning, and a 4- to 13-millimeter "drop" (the height difference between heel and toe). For a complete shoe guide, visit twopct.com/p/ruckingshoe.

## HOW TO ADJUST THE STRAPS OF YOUR PACK

As we learned earlier, you want the weight close to and somewhat high on your back. The straps on your backpack can help you achieve this. If they're too loose, the weight will sit lower on your body. At the same time, if the straps are too tight, they can rub the inside of your shoulders.

Adjust them in a way that feels most comfortable as you're walking. The pack shouldn't feel like it's hanging too low on your back, but it also should not feel as tight as a straitjacket. In general, the pack should be an inch or two below where your neck and back meet.

Also remember that you can and should adjust the straps as you walk. If your shoulders become uncomfortable, tightening or loosening the shoulder straps can shift the load and make your walk more comfortable. You can even hang the pack or vest off one shoulder for a little while, then shift it to the other shoulder. These techniques can help you cover more miles.

Some backpacks also have sternum straps that run across your chest, and hip belts that wrap around your waist. We'll cover those in the next chapter.

## KEEP YOUR OWN PACE

We carry weight so infrequently today that tossing a weight on our back can be a bit jarring. Your body will seem to ask you, "*What* are you doing?"

This is why I recommend people start walking at their normal pace. Use your initial walks to get familiar with having weight on your back. Don't worry about pushing yourself too fast—yet. After you've walked with weight a handful of times and your body begins to get it, you can begin to push the pace.

Most people intuitively know when they're walking faster than normal. But one way to ensure that you are, in fact, walking faster is to track a normal walk on a GPS app like Strava. It'll tell you what your average mile time is. So simply use a GPS app to track a regular walk and then use the app again when you want to increase your pace—your mile time should be lower.

Keep in mind, however, that your mile times might change if you change your route. For example, if you compared a flat route to a hilly route, your time on the hilly route would probably be slower even if you were working physically harder.

## BE MINDFUL OF YOUR POSTURE

Since we were kids, we have always been told to "stand up straight." Standing straight allows us to walk and run more efficiently compared to if we are leaning back or slumped over. So you might think you must stand perfectly upright as you walk with weight.

In practice, however, having weight on your back changes your posture. A study in the journal *Ergonomics* found that when people put a weighted pack on their back, they lean slightly forward to counter the weight. That natural forward lean helps you find a stronger center of gravity. It also leads your core to work harder, strengthening it.

So don't worry if you lean forward a bit when you walk. That's normal. At the same time, you should only be leaning forward a few degrees. If you must lean forward more than that, you should probably use a lighter weight in the pack.

That same study found that weighted vests led to a more upright posture, so you might think that wearing a weighted vest is optimal, but it's actually more complicated than that. We'll cover the differences between walking with weighted packs and vests in chapter 8.

## HOW OFTEN AND FAR SHOULD I WALK AT FIRST?

The beauty of walking with weight is that it's something you can do every day. If ancient humans couldn't walk with weight every single day, we'd have all died off, because carrying weight was necessary for survival.

That said, when you are just starting, use lighter weights or give yourself some time between days you walk with weight. For example, if you walk with weight 2 days in a row, consider walking without weight on the third day. Having days off during your first month of walking with weight gives your body time to recover and adapt.

Distance-wise, use your normal walks as a guide. If you typically walk, say, 3 miles around your neighborhood, use that same distance in your initial walks. You don't want your first walks to be significantly longer than your body is used to. Easing in allows your body to adequately adapt—it keeps you in the sweet spot of improving fitness but not pushing yourself into the red.

# 6

# LEVEL UP

Once you've mastered the basics outlined in the last chapter and made walking with weight part of your regular (or semi-regular) routine, you'll start to really experience the overall benefits and you may be ready to level up.

Just like with any workout, when walking with weight, there are myriad ways to increase your fitness level and improve your strength. The tactics in this chapter will help you by exploring:

- Four ways to increase the intensity.
- Why you probably shouldn't run while wearing a weighted pack or vest.
- The heaviest weight you should walk with.
- The benefits of sternum straps and hip belts on backpacks.
- How to set goals.
- Why you should make weighted walking as easy as possible.

You'll enhance your routine and achieve better results by leaning into these tactics. Understanding or implementing each will teach you to walk with weight stronger and faster so you can expand your health, fitness, and what you're capable of.

## INCREASE THE INTENSITY

There are four straightforward ways to make walking with weight more challenging to increase your health and performance:

1. **Increase the load:** Add more weight to your pack or vest.
2. **Increase your pace:** Walk faster.
3. **Increase the distance:** Walk farther.
4. **Vary the terrain:** Walk steeper hills and uneven ground.

But first let's quickly cover how to think about improvement.

We live in a society where we always think that more, faster, and stronger are better. But we forget that reaching more, faster, and stronger comes with a trade-off: To reach peak fitness, you must exercise significantly more. That extra exercise indeed improves your health and fitness, but you can hit a rate of diminishing returns. Once you get fit and healthy, becoming even more fit and healthy takes even more work.

For example, a person who takes just 2,500 steps a day significantly reduces their risk of disease if they begin taking 5,000 steps a day. One review of the research published in *Preventive Medicine* found that going from 2,500 to 5,000 steps a day could decrease your risk of all-cause mortality by about a third. That's significant. Just 2,500 extra steps—the equivalent of about 20 extra minutes of moving across a day—are extremely powerful for someone who's rather inactive.

But those same 2,500 steps aren't as powerful for someone who's already highly active. For example, that same review in *Preventive Medicine* found that the health benefits of extra steps are negligible beyond about 12,500 a day. That means going from 12,500 to 15,000 steps a day doesn't seem to improve your (already good) health all that much further. You might get a boost of a percent or two.

### Ideal steps per day

One *Two Percent* reader asked me, "How many steps a day is best?"

I wish I could give a hard-and-fast number. But there's some uncertainty in the science. For example, one study in *JAMA* found that the women with the lowest risk of all-cause mortality (death by any cause) got in 7,500 or more steps a day. Interestingly enough, those who got in far more than 7,500 steps weren't any better off.

Then again, another study in *JAMA* found that getting 8,000 steps per day led to a 51 percent lower risk of all-cause mortality compared to getting 4,000. Which is good—but not as good as getting in 12,000 steps per day. The people who hit that number had a 65 percent lower risk. So *that* study suggests that more is better. But the catch, as we can see in the study, is that there is a diminishing return.

My take, after reading all the data, is this: A bare minimum for health is probably around 7,500 steps per day. But if you have enough time and want to be extra careful, get in at least 12,000 steps daily.

And as you rack up more steps, don't lose sight of the larger goal. We don't just walk to avoid disease. We do it to live better. I try to go on a walk every single day. It's not just for the steps—it's for unplugged time outside to clear my head. I probably won't see any possible reduction of disease risk benefits from these walks until I'm old. But I can get a physical and mental boost right now, with each step.

In fact, walking much beyond that can present its own challenges. For example, you'll likely spend less time on other practices and responsibilities that can improve your life. Every healthy behavior hits a rate of diminishing returns. Keep that in mind.

And one quick word of warning before we begin: One reader of my Substack *Two Percent*, Olivia, had perhaps the simplest and wisest words about how to level up and improve your fitness sustainably. She wrote: "The main tip I have for improvement is to not increase the weight, pace, or distance at the same time. Do one at a time."

Her tip works by not overloading us with too much, too soon. By increasing just one parameter at a time, you can focus on improvement in that one area and prevent overdoing it.

## INCREASE THE LOAD

When it comes to the weight of your pack or vest, more isn't always better. I've found that consistently walking with between 10 and 20 percent of your body weight is a sustainable target.

If we go significantly under 10 percent, we miss out on some benefits. If we go over 20 percent, the act can start to become uncomfortable to the point that we may walk a shorter distance. If you use too much weight, the act of walking with weight starts to become the opposite of fun—and you'll probably not only walk shorter distances but will also go less often.

**The lesson:** Using a weight that feels uncomfortable but not despair-inducing will make the act more enjoyable and allow you to get in more miles. If you do that, you'll probably end up walking much farther, leading you to burn more total calories compared with if you walked a shorter distance with a heavier load.

For instance, let's say walking 1 mile with 25 pounds burns 140 calories per mile, but walking with 50 pounds burns 180 calories per mile. Over that mile, you'd burn more calories carrying 50 pounds instead of 25. What tends to happen in the real world, however, is that people end up walking more miles using a lighter weight, leading them to burn more calories overall. With 50 pounds, you might walk 2 miles and burn 360 calories. But with 25 pounds, you might walk 4 miles, leading you to burn 560—or 200 extra calories.

The goal is to find a weight that allows you to balance both strength and endurance—not too heavy that you don't go far, but not so light that you don't get a strength stimulus.

This is why I usually walk with about 35 pounds, or around 20 percent of my body weight. That weight is challenging yet sustainable for a longer distance. It gives me a great fitness boost but makes my walks more enjoyable.

Of course, I sometimes walk with more than that if I have

a good reason. For example, if I'm preparing for a long backpacking trip or backcountry hunt, I might train with a heavier weight leading up to my outdoor trip. Or I might be crunched for time and want to do as much physical work as possible in my limited schedule.

Sometimes I'll go lighter than 30 pounds. My wife, Leah, and I, for example, typically take a long walk together every Saturday morning. We'll walk to a coffee shop anywhere from 4 to 7 miles away, grab a coffee, then walk home, giving us an 8- to 14-mile walk. It's my favorite time of the week—an opportunity for us to connect and reflect.

I'll typically use 20 pounds on those walks. I find that after about 7 miles of walking with my regular 30 pounds, the walk starts to feel more like a legitimate workout—and that takes away from our conversations.

I believe I'm more holistically healthy by finding the balance between making the walk a bit more challenging but not so challenging that I can't reap the many benefits of human connection.

## INCREASE YOUR PACE

Once you've started walking at your normal pace, walking faster is a great way to elevate your heart rate and get more endurance benefits from walking with weight. It may also help you live longer.

Research consistently shows a strong relationship between walking speed and your risk of various diseases—heart disease, cognitive decline, and more. For example:

- Researchers at Harvard and Boston University, during a decade-long study, found that men in their sixties who could walk 4 miles an hour (a 15-minute mile) instead of just 2 miles an hour were 13 percent less likely to die.

- A study in *PLOS One* discovered that people aged 50 to 72 who were the faster walkers of the study were 87 percent less at risk of heart disease.
- The trend holds true for younger people, too. University of Sydney researchers sampled 50,000 people of all ages and found those who could walk at least 3 miles an hour were 20 percent less at risk of all-cause mortality. The fastest walkers saw an extra bump—their risk decreased by 24 percent.

So it pays to be able to walk briskly.

In the last chapter, we covered how most people intuitively know when they're walking faster. Still, tools like Strava, Garmin, or any other GPS app or device can help us.

If you don't want to be even more tethered to tech, you can determine your pace with phone-free methods. Use something as simple as the clock on your microwave. Let's say you walk the same route twice. If one walk takes you 60 minutes but the other takes you 55 minutes, you walked faster on that second walk.

When it comes to increasing your pace, ease in. Try to decrease your mile times 20 to 30 seconds at a time. That might seem like a lot if you're a runner, but remember that walking is a much slower act. If you go from walking a 20-minute mile to a 19:40 mile, that's about a 2 percent increase in pace.

Aim to drop your pace by 20 to 30 seconds every week or two, settling into a brisk pace. The data suggests walking 4 miles an hour—the equivalent of a 15-minute per mile pace on a flat surface—is a great goal to shoot for. That's a 4-miles-an-hour pace. Research shows hitting that pace reduces our risk of many health issues.

You can even mix in different paces. For example, you could walk 1 mile at an average pace, then push yourself the next mile, then drop back down to an average pace for a third mile.

### Walk, don't run

As we covered earlier in the book, running was critical to human evolution. Ancient humans were "essentially professional athletes whose livelihood required them to be physically active," one Harvard anthropologist told me. To stay alive, early humans had to be very physically versatile. They were capable at just about every physical skill, from movement to endurance to strength.

On the other hand, modern people in the developed world sit an average of 9 to 10 hours a day. Our inactive lifestyles give us weird muscle weaknesses, strength imbalances, and restricted movement patterns.

We're also heavier people than we were in the past. For example, the average modern hunter-gatherer, who scientists believe is an accurate representation of an ancient human, weighs around 125 pounds, while the average modern American man and woman weigh 200 and 170 pounds, respectively.

Collectively, this means that when we run, we do so with our wonky movement patterns, weaknesses, and heavier bodies. This likely explains why, if you recall the study from chapter 3, "27% to 70% of recreational and competitive distance runners sustain an overuse running injury during any 1-year period." Adding weight to running increases a person's injury risk further.

A group of scientists at the University of Wisconsin studied this exact topic and found that running with a 20-pound weight vest was potentially harmful. They found that it led to force changes that would likely bring about the condition of runner's knee relatively quicker.

Of course, plenty of people run a couple of miles with a 20-pound vest during the popular Memorial Day Murph Challenge—a workout where you run a mile, then do 100 pull-ups, 200 push-ups, 300 squats, and run another mile all while wearing a weight vest. Their knees don't spontaneously combust afterward. So, you'll probably be fine if you do it now and then, but I would keep the weight around 5 percent of your body weight or less and wouldn't make it a regular part of your routine.

If you want or need to ruck faster, try to speed walk. It's faster than a walk but slower than a run, where one foot is always maintaining ground contact. That will allow you to achieve a quick pace without hammering your knees.

## INCREASE THE DISTANCE

Just like with weight and pace, ease into longer distances. Once you've started walking with weight and found a distance that feels challenging but doable, slowly add more distance.

Increase your walks by a half mile or so to start. Remember, the number one cause of injury in any physical activity is doing too much too quickly. I'd rather you ease into adding miles than tackle too many too soon and get an ache that leads you to have to take a couple weeks off.

## VARY THE TERRAIN

Using trails can be a fun way to boost the intensity and benefits of your walks. Trails offer far more challenges than a sidewalk: more ups and downs, looser ground, more obstacles, more to pay attention to.

Biomechanists at the University of Michigan discovered that the increased challenge of walking or running on rough, uneven trails leads people to burn 28 percent more energy per step. That bears repeating: 28 percent.

Of course, that figure is a generality. A tame, flat trail would likely out-edge a flat road by, say, 12 percent. That's according to a small study published in the *Journal of Sports Science and Medicine*. But a rough, up-and-down trail might push us to burn perhaps 50 to 100 percent more calories per step.

Trails may also work our muscles harder. One study noted, "[Trails] tend to invoke higher challenges for the neuromuscular system, especially regarding involved muscle coordination, proprioception, and activation compared to [roads]." It's likely why one study found trail runners generally have stronger lower bodies than road runners.

What's more—and this is the most interesting to me—is that you may get more brain benefits from being on a trail.

Exercise benefits our brains. This we know. It seems to increase the volume of areas of the brain associated with memory and thinking. But not all exercise is equally brain-building. If walking on a sidewalk is like addition and subtraction, walking on a trail is more like multivariable calculus.

"When you combine physical acts with cognitive acts, it tends to have a really beneficial effect on the brain," researchers at USC told me.

To understand this, consider my experience walking with weight on a sidewalk versus in the deserts around my home.

On a sidewalk, I can just zone out and go where the sidewalk takes me.

A trail, on the other hand, forces mental engagement. The rocky ground makes me play something like moving Tetris as I walk. With each step, I must quickly angle and land my feet in slits of flat ground between serrated rocks, pivot on loose dirt, sidestep spiny cacti, or hurdle tiny cliffs.

Each step is new, and nothing is preprogrammed. I have to quickly consider so many variables, such as:

- How should I pace myself?
- Should I hammer up this hill, or will that lead me to bonk later on?
- If I bomb a downhill section, how should I position my body and pace myself relative to the slope of the hill, given that it's covered in loose dirt?
- How should I angle my foot as I walk through a patch of rocks?
- Are there agave or cacti hanging onto the trail that could cut me?

If I zone out, I'll be hobbling home on a twisted ankle or eating schist.

The scientists believe this mental engagement as we

move could help us fend off age-related brain diseases like Alzheimer's.

## WHAT'S THE MAXIMUM WEIGHT I CAN USE?

As I've already mentioned, walking with between 10 and 20 percent of your body weight is a great go-to weight. You can lessen the load if you're going significantly farther, or you can add more weight if you have a good reason.

Some people, however, want to go as heavy as possible. They ask me some variation of the question "What's the heaviest weight I can use and still stay safe?"

I've looked at military research spanning centuries. Much of it suggests we shouldn't go over 50 pounds. Fifty pounds is the heaviest load that allows soldiers to fight like hell, stay injury-free, and forge elite strength and performance. That's according to research going back to the 1800s, which was recently reaffirmed by three different studies from the US Army, Navy, and Marines.

But there's a problem: All that research was conducted on male soldiers. These soldiers tend to be generally larger people with similar body types. That means that the 50-pound rule doesn't apply to people who aren't built like soldiers. For example, walking with 50 pounds is experienced differently by someone who weighs 110 pounds versus someone who weighs 220 pounds. That weight might be far too much for the smaller person.

Research supports this: In 1950, Colonel S. L. A. Marshall did scores of studies on walking with weight. He concluded that a pack weighing the equivalent of one-third your body weight is the heaviest you should ever use.

He wasn't recommending the weight; rather, he was telling the military they shouldn't ask their soldiers to march with more than one-third their body weight. Regularly going above that weight, Colonel Marshall found, increases your risk of injury and impedes your ability to move well.

To use our examples above, a 180-pound person wouldn't want to regularly walk with more than 70 pounds. A 110-pound person wouldn't want to exceed 35 pounds.

**How much weight should I use if I'm overweight?**

The question of how much weight to use if you're in the overweight or obese category based on BMI is critically important. More than 70 percent of Americans are overweight or obese and, as we learned, walking with weight is arguably the best exercise to help people lose weight because it preferentially burns fat while preserving muscle. That can lead to better long-term health outcomes.

But if you're overweight or obese, it may be confusing to figure out how much weight you should use based on your body weight. For example, if you weigh 300 pounds and start with 15 percent of your body weight, that suggests you should use 45 pounds. That may be too heavy because much of that 300 pounds is likely from fat and is not actually helping support the weight.

So how do we account for the fact that body weight guidelines are useful for individualizing weight, but also that they might be useless (even dangerous) for a significant number of people?

**My conclusion:** Err on the side of using less weight than the body weight guidelines suggest—the more overweight you are, the more you'll want to take away from what the guidelines suggest. Experiment. Use a weight that feels heavy but doable. If your first walks feel miserable, use less weight.

## SHOULD YOU EVER USE YOUR "HEAVIEST WEIGHT"?

Using a heavy weight—one-third of your body weight—for a relatively shorter walk from time to time can be a fun challenge. As long as you don't go too far or do it too often, you may benefit from the occasional heavy walk.

For example, one study on soldiers found that an occasional heavy walk increased fitness and didn't lead to injuries. But it also found that problems tend to arise when we do multiple heavy walks multiple days in a row. The stress on the body and lack of recovery push us into the red. This is one reason why walking with weight has a higher injury rate in the military than it does among the general population. The military often has soldiers marching with very heavy loads for days on end.

## USE A STERNUM STRAP AND HIP BELT

Many backpacks have sternum straps and hip belts.

The sternum strap is the smaller strap that latches to the front of the shoulder straps and runs across your chest.

This strap isn't just to keep the pack on your body; it can help spread the weight of the pack across your chest and take pressure off your shoulders. Try using the sternum strap if your pack has one. Experiment and find what works best for you.

A hip belt is the belt attached to the pack's bottom that, you guessed it, secures around your hips. Hip belts are especially beneficial and allow you to distribute some of the pack's weight to your much stronger hips instead of having all the weight ride entirely on your shoulders.

One study in the *Journal of Biomechanics* found, "Carrying a heavy backpack with a hip belt results in reduced shoulder forces, spinal forces, activation of the [shoulder] muscles, as well as increased comfort for the carrier and improved performance on selected tasks when compared to a backpack with no hip belt."

I've realized the value of hip belts, especially while walking with heavy packs in the outdoors.

When my pack gets heavy, I'll walk for about 15 minutes with the weight riding mostly on the shoulder straps. Eventually, however, those shoulder straps can feel like they are trying to slice me lengthwise into thirds, so I'll pull the hip belt tight and loosen the shoulder straps, allowing the weight to ride mostly on my hips.

After another 15 minutes, my lower body muscles begin to feel like they're being burned off my body, so I'll then do something in between, where the weight is equally distributed between the belt and shoulder straps. It's exceedingly helpful, and I even use a hip belt on my daily walks.

Some thinkers in the world of walking with weight don't recommend hip belts. But when I polled readers of my newsletter, *Two Percent*, the most common tip was to use a hip belt.

One reader, Steve, wrote, "I've walked with and without a hip belt. The hip belt seems to help with overall weight placement and comfort." Another reader, Diane, wrote, "Having a hip belt was so important, especially as I increased the weight. The hip belt allowed me to shift where the weight sat on my body, especially over long periods. That helped me walk farther."

My advice: If your pack has a hip belt, use it and see if it helps you.

I've also discovered two other amazing features of the hip belt:

- I thread the belt through my dogs' leash handles. The leashes are then attached to the belt, which frees my hands when I walk my dogs. This actually makes walking my dogs even more comfortable than if I weren't wearing a weighted pack. I can walk more naturally than if I were holding leashes and even send an email or two if I have to.
- Some readers of *Two Percent* mentioned their bags have small accessory pockets on the hip belt that allow them to keep their phone and a snack at the ready. This is why we added built-in hip belts with pockets to our packs from WalkFully (more on that in the chapter 8).

A few people have asked me where they should place the hip belt. My first (sarcastic) thought was "on your hips." But I learned that some backpackers say your hip belt should be up high, resting at the very top of your hip bones and above your belly button. This backpacking ideology, naturally, has trickled into the circles of people who walk with weight for exercise.

The thing about backpackers, though, is that they generally try to have the lightest pack possible. Many Appalachian Trail hikers, for example, use a pack that weighs less than 10 pounds, not including food and water. I've even heard of ultralight backpackers cutting half the handle off their toothbrush just to save half an ounce.

People who walk with weight, on the other hand, embrace the weight. Our packs are heavy for the sake of being heavy. This is why backpacking rules don't always apply to walking with weight and won't necessarily help us meet our fitness goals.

I pondered the placement question and read the research. My conclusion: Don't overthink the belt placement. I just cinch it where it feels most natural at any given time. Usually that's lower on my hips, because if the belt is high and tight, it can impact my ability to breathe freely. But I don't think there's one "magic spot."

## SET GOALS

Goals are good for us: Research shows that fitness goals improve our motivation to exercise, adhere to a workout plan, and, in turn, improve our health. But we need to set the right goals.

New research shows the key is to set goals that are specific and that challenge us. Those goals lead to bigger performance gains than goals that are too easy or vague. And that makes sense: A specific goal gives you a clear target, and if that target is harder to achieve, you must increase your capabilities to reach it.

For example, "Walk 5 miles with 20 pounds in my pack by April 1" is better than "Walk farther with more weight."

Need a goal? In chapter 10, we'll explain five amazing challenges the military has used to prepare its soldiers. We've adapted each to varying ability levels.

## MAKE IT EASY

Years of psychological research show that we're more likely to do things that are easier to do. Here are a few stats about this I love:

- Slot machine usage more than doubled when casinos removed the clunky handles and swapped them with buttons. The handles required gamblers to physically pull the handle downward a foot or two every game. "SPIN" buttons, on the other hand, take only a tap. The ease of these buttons led slot gaming rates to go from roughly 400 games an hour to 900 games an hour.
- Online retailers who remove steps to buy a product increase their sales conversions by anywhere from 50 to 100 percent.
- One junk food executive told me that the key to the rise of junk food was what he called "velocity." The food industry designed junk food to be quicker and easier to eat—it requires no preparation and is easier to chew and swallow—and that set off its meteoric rise in the 1970s.

Today, many corporations try to make things as easy as possible so we'll buy more, eat more, gamble more, and do more of other behaviors that can hurt us in the long run. But here's some good news: We can also use this phenomenon to do more things that help us.

Readers of my *Two Percent* Substack have found this phenomenon to be especially true when it comes to walking with weight.

- Sherry, a high-level executive and dog mom, wrote, “Putting my weighted pack right by my dog’s leash makes me wear my pack when I walk my dog every day.”
- Terry, a retiree in Florida, wrote, “I leave my pack by the front door so I see it and use it more often.”
- Maryann, a busy mom, wrote, “I prep my pack the night before my morning walk. It saves me lots of time getting out the door.”
- Dale, who works for the Bureau of Land Management in the field, keeps a weighted pack in his work truck. When he has down time or long waits at different job sites, he tosses it on and goes for a stroll.

I do the same. I keep a pack and three different-size weights on my back porch. When I take my dogs for a walk, I see the pack and remember to take it. Behavioral science for the win!

# 7

# SUPPORT

Throughout the years, I've discovered numerous tips and strategies on a variety of topics that help us walk with weight better. Some deal in nutrition—for example, hydration and nutrition while walking with weight. Others bolster your body so you can perform better and reach your peak performance. Some may seem minor, but I've learned that the little things can mean a lot. Thus, in this chapter I'll cover some additional, helpful advice I believe can make your walk or workout as effective as possible.

## *STAY HYDRATED*

Around 275 BC, Erasistratus of Ceos became the first physician to think seriously about water intake, sweat, and health. By the 1800s, we realized how crucial the balance of salt and water is to our overall well-being. Today, we know hydration isn't just about water; it's also about maintaining key electrolytes—sodium, potassium, magnesium, and chloride—that keep us performing at our best.

When we walk with weight, especially in the heat, we often lose water and electrolytes through sweat. Dehydration sets in when we lose more fluid than we replace, typically becoming noticeable once we drop about 2 percent of our body weight in water. For a 150-pound person, that's roughly 3 pounds or 48 ounces of water. Early signs of dehydration include fatigue, dizziness, and reduced focus and coordination. Severe dehydration can lead to heat stroke, kidney issues, seizures, or shock.

Now that I've terrified you with a death warning, here's some reassuring news: Research shows that dehydration is uncommon for most healthy adults with easy access to clean water. Unless you're engaging in extreme endurance events, performing labor-intensive tasks in high heat, or lack access to clean water, dehydration isn't typically a major concern.

For regular workouts lasting up to 90 minutes, drinking water before your walk should suffice. You probably don't need electrolyte supplements, because most people get plenty of electrolytes through their normal diet.

If you exercise longer than that or if it's particularly hot outside, nutrition expert Mike Roussell, PhD, suggests you take water and consistently drink small amounts rather than waiting to get thirsty. You may also want to use electrolyte supplements. That ensures your body effectively absorbs and uses the water you consume.

Here's a simple two-step hydration strategy backed by science:

**Step 1: Start hydrated.** Research indicates many athletes begin activities slightly dehydrated, which can hurt their performance. In the 24 hours before an event or rigorous workout, hydrate consistently. Let your pee guide you: "Aim for a light straw color in your urine as a simple gauge of hydration status," said Roussell. If your pee looks like highlighter marker fluid, you need more water.

**Step 2: Drink according to thirst.** Forget rigid rules like 8 glasses daily—hydration needs vary widely. Drinking according to thirst is effective for most people. Drink a little more if you're exercising more than 90 minutes, where thirst cues can become less reliable. In these cases, regularly sipping water is ideal. Consider electrolyte supplements if it's hot out.

Ultimately, hydration doesn't need to be complicated. Start your activity hydrated, sip consistently, and let your thirst—and your urine color—guide you.

## FUEL YOUR WALKS

We tend to overcomplicate sports nutrition, thinking that eating a special food will radically enhance our fitness. What's more, we have an entire sports nutrition complex pushing energy bars and goos on us and claiming their expensive products will make us perform better.

Most everyday people, however, don't need to get in the weeds about sports nutrition. Instead, understanding a few key principles can help you fuel your walks.

For most people, a casual walk with a weighted vest or weighted pack doesn't require special nutrition. Your body has enough stored energy from your last meal to get you through at least 60 minutes of walking with weight, and probably even longer. Here's what you should do:

- **Before the walk:** Eat a regular meal or snack with some protein and carbohydrates 1 to 3 hours before heading out. Something like Greek yogurt with fruit, a banana with peanut butter, or eggs and toast work well.
- **During the walk:** You likely don't need to eat anything unless you're walking for much longer than an hour.
- **After the walk:** If you're hungry, eat a balanced meal with protein, healthy fats, and carbs to replenish your energy and aid recovery.

If you're using walking with weight as a tool to aid weight loss, keep in mind that the number one rule you must follow is to eat fewer calories than you're burning over a day. For weight loss, focus on nutrition. It's really hard to lose weight through exercise alone. It takes *a lot* of exercise to lose weight.

That said, walking with weight might be one of the best exercises you can do as you overhaul your diet and lose weight. It will help you burn some calories and force more of your weight loss to come from fat—preserving more muscle and improving your health.

Here are some tips to follow if you're trying to lose weight:

- **Before exercise:** Have a light meal or snack if needed, but keep it minimal to avoid unnecessary calorie intake.
- **During exercise:** Skip the energy bars and sports drinks unless you're exercising intensely for more than 90 minutes. Most people have plenty of stored energy to fuel most walks.

- **After exercise:** Avoid overcompensating. If weight loss is your goal, ensure that you don't eat back all the calories you burned. Stick to a balanced postworkout meal and monitor your food intake.
- **Over the course of the day:** Try to eat protein with each meal, as that may help you preserve muscle mass as you lose weight.

## DO THIS SIMPLE WARMUP

Most people skip warmups. I get it. Warmups are no fun, and many take too long. Yet when I sent out the survey about walking with weight to readers of my Substack, *Two Percent*, many people mentioned that a quick pre-walk warmup helped them feel better during and after the walk.

One reader said they "swore by" a quick stretching session before walking. Another said, "I do a 5-minute warmup before I leave. Once I started doing this, I stopped having discomfort after really long rucks." Yet another said, "Warming up my shoulders has helped me avoid stiffness in my neck and shoulders when I'm walking with weight."

Many pointed to a warmup I'd published a year earlier, called the Two Percent Warmup, as their go-to.

We need it now more than ever because many of us sit a significant portion of the day, leading to tighter muscles and poor movement. When we exercise with those stiff muscles and odd movement patterns, we're more likely to feel some discomfort after any activity. What's more, moving better can also help unlock new performance, allowing you to push your fitness and become healthier.

The good news is, shorter warmups are often better.

Research shows that excessively long warmups can actually decrease your performance. On the other hand, quick and dynamic warmups get you ready to go.

## The Two Percent Warmup

I first shared this warmup on my *Two Percent* Substack—and readers loved it. It helped them perform better during the workout and feel better after it. It also helped them heal nagging injuries and avoid future ones.

The warmup takes fewer than 10 minutes, and I even look forward to it. It's a calm, quiet moment of every day. I provide details below on why the exercises work and instructions on how to perform them correctly. To see videos of the exercises, scan the QR code on page 113.

1. **Couch Stretch**
   This exercise helps you extend your hips and stretches your quads, which can become tight from walking with weight, running, and cycling. In fact, Kelly and Juliett Starrett, physical therapists and two of the brightest minds in performance and injury prevention, say that being able to extend your hips "may have the biggest impact on your everyday functionality."
   **How to do it:** Kneel facing away from a wall. Pin your right knee between the floor and the wall, your right shin running up the wall. Now move your left leg forward and place your foot on the ground. You should be in a lunge position, with your left leg forward and left knee bent 90 degrees, your right leg back with your shin running up the wall. Hold the position and squeeze your butt. You should feel the stretch in your right quad. If you've never done this stretch, you'll be tight and may be unable

to get into the position. In that case, stabilize yourself by holding on to something.

**Reps:** Hold the stretch for 1 minute on your right leg, then switch legs and repeat on your left leg.

2. **Plank Walk-Up**

   Many of us have relatively immobile ankles and upper backs. Thanks, desk work! That can throw off our ability to squat, lunge, pick up stuff from the ground, lift stuff overhead, and more. The result is that we're more likely to injure our shoulders, neck, low back, and hips.

   This exercise mobilizes your ankles and upper back while improving your breathing.

   **How to do it:** Get into a push-up position. Now walk your feet toward your hands while keeping your legs straight, your hips rising. Keep your arms straight. Once you can't walk any closer to your hands without your legs bending, hold the stretch, breathe deeply, and "pedal" your heels toward the ground. You should feel the stretch down the backside of your body, especially in your calves.

   **Reps:** Walk into the position and "pedal" your heels toward the ground 50 times each. It should take you about 30 to 45 seconds.

3. **Modified Hip Pigeon**

   People generally favor their right side when they stand, shifting their weight into their right hip. That causes your left hip to become tight because it rarely moves through a full range of motion. (Fun fact: Even left-handed people tend to shift to their right hip when they stand.)

   If you don't move often, your tight left hip may never cause you any real issues. Once you add exercise to an imbalanced lower body, however, you set yourself up for problems. This stretch unwinds and balances your hips.

**How to do it:** Get on all fours and place your left knee on top of a foam roller, yoga brick, or rolled-up towel so it's elevated. Now extend your right leg and cross it over your left leg. Your right leg should now be on the left side of your left leg. From this position, push your hips leftward in a pulsing motion. You should feel the stretch in your left hip.
**Reps:** Stretch 1 minute on your left side to start. As your left side becomes more mobile, begin performing the stretch on your right side as well.

4. **Kneeling Overhead Kettlebell Windmill**

This exercise is like a combo meal—a lot of good in one package. It builds your overhead strength and range of motion while forcing you to control your shoulder in a vulnerable position. It also strengthens your core and improves your ability to rotate and move your hips (people today rarely "twist").

The result: You'll be better at everything and have a stronger core; more resilient shoulders; less back, hip, knee pain; and so on.

**How to do it:** Get in the lunge position with your right leg forward and a kettlebell or your weighted pack in front of you. Grab the weight with your right hand and press it overhead so it's hanging behind your wrist. This is the start. Now slowly twist your torso as you bring it down toward the ground. Touch your left elbow to the ground, then return to the start. You should feel this in your hips. Do all your reps, then repeat on your other side. It may take you a while to be able to tap the ground with your elbow, so use very light weights to start and ease in.
**Reps:** 4 to 8 on each side.

5. **Half-Moon Stretch**

   This stretches your back, shoulders, and hips before you place weight on your back and torso.

   **How to do it:** Stand tall. Bring your arms vertically overhead and straight. Clasp your hands together. Now push your hips leftward and your hands rightward, making a big "half-moon" shape with your body. You should feel the stretch in your left side. Hold it for a couple of seconds. Now repeat on the other side. Go back and forth.

   **Reps:** 5 to 10 on each side.

6. **Side Lunge Stretch**

   This one opens up your hip adductor muscles. These muscles stabilize your pelvis when you walk with weight. When they're tight, it can lead to knee, hip, or low back pain and generally inefficient walking and running.

   **How to do it:** Stand tall and spread your feet about 2 or 3 times hips' width apart. Bend your right knee and drop your hips, lowering yourself into a side lunge to the right. Keep your left leg straight. You should feel the stretch on the inside of your left leg. Sit into the stretch for a moment so you really feel it. Stand up and repeat on your left side.

   **Reps:** 5 to 10 on each side.

You can find a detailed video of each of the Two Percent Warmup exercises to help with proper form and execution by scanning the following QR code:

## KEEP YOUR SHOULDERS HAPPY

Since writing *The Comfort Crisis*, I've received many messages that sound something like this: "I read your book and started rucking, but my shoulders sometimes ache while I'm walking with my pack. Do you have any advice for me?"

To find the best and safest advice, I spoke to Dr. Doug Kechijian. Doug is a doctor of physical therapy who often treats military personnel, and he was a member of the Special Forces as a pararescueman, which means he's thought deeply about walking with weight and has done a lot himself.

He told me that as long as you stay within smart weight recommendations—using 10 to 30 percent of your body weight—it's unlikely you'll injure your shoulders while rucking.

"Most people are not really in true pain shoulder-wise after walking with a weighted pack," Doug said. "It's more like discomfort. I think discomfort in the shoulders is relatively normal. You have straps digging into your shoulders and a long duration of compressive loading on them, no matter how well you fitted your ruck. This isn't bad per se, and your body adapts. But it is fatiguing."

Research backs this up. Scientists in the United Kingdom took a bunch of young military recruits who hadn't walked with weight and had them march with a 45-pound pack on a fast-moving incline treadmill for 2 hours straight. The result: 90 percent of the participants reported shoulder discomfort.

Which, duh. Doing anything new for 2 hours straight can cause discomfort. If you asked me to handwrite letters for 2 hours straight, I'd report hand discomfort. I'd also report butt and back discomfort if I sat at a writing desk for 2 hours straight.

The study isn't surprising—but it can explain why your shoulders might hurt when you walk with weight.

When we do something physical that our body isn't used to—in our case, walking with a heavier weight or longer than usual—it uses the sensations of discomfort and pain to basically ask us, "WTF are you doing right now?" It's a sort of smoke alarm letting us know that there's a chance that what we're doing could become problematic.

But, as with real smoke alarms, there's usually no fire. At the same time, ignoring a smoke alarm is not wise. Doug said, "Typically, discomfort can be a warning of some kind that needs to be heeded."

The good news is there's a simple fix for shoulder discomfort: Hang from a pull-up bar. Why? The weight of rucking compresses your shoulders. "Hanging essentially does the opposite," Doug said. "It's lengthening, so it works as a nice reset." It's such a radical change in the area that it turns the smoke alarm off.

There are different ways to hang and get the most benefit. Try these three:

1. **Dead hang:** Just hang from a bar with both of your arms extended straight overhead, ideally at a height where your feet clear the ground, for at least 30 seconds, breathing in and out deeply.
2. **Hang with a swing.** Hang vertically from a bar with both of your arms extended straight overhead, keeping your body relaxed. You should feel a stretch in your shoulders. Now slightly swing side to side. Swing 10 to 20 times in each direction.
3. **Monkey hang:** Hang from a bar with both arms extended straight overhead. Now let go with your right hand briefly so you slightly swing leftward. Grab the bar again, then repeat with your left arm. Repeat. Do

that 5 to 10 times on each hand, depending on your grip strength.

You can find a detailed video of each of these hangs to help with proper form and execution by scanning the following QR code:

## PROTECT YOUR KNEES

Knee pains are very common—they hit people who exercise often and those who sit often. They're especially prevalent in people who run and to a much lesser extent in people who walk with weight and cycle.

One solution to knee pain—in addition to doing the Couch Stretch in the Two Percent Warmup we just covered—is to strengthen all the muscles around your knees.

The best version of this exercise requires a quad extension machine, available at most gyms. Sit in the machine, select an appropriate weight, then—with your right leg only—move your leg just a few degrees out so it's bearing weight. You should feel your quad working. Hold that static position for 30 seconds. Repeat with your other leg. Do that for as many as 3 sets.

If you don't have access to a quad extension machine, no problem. Get in the lunge position and hold it for 30 seconds on each leg. Do that for as many as 3 sets.

## BOLSTER YOUR BACK

In chapter 3, we covered how walking with weight can help prevent and relieve back pain. And that's important. Up to 80 percent of people experience low back pain at some point in their life, and 25 percent of people have had back pain in the last few months. What's more, people with chronic low back pain are twice as likely to suffer from depression, anxiety, psychosis, and sleep deprivation.

Preventing and relieving back pain is a key benefit of walking with weight. But you can make your back even stronger and more bulletproof with three exercises from Dr. Stuart McGill. McGill is arguably the world's foremost authority on back pain. He has studied the topic for decades and has racked up tens of thousands of citations from other researchers.

He's discovered three particularly effective exercises for preventing and rehabilitating back pain and has used them to help everyone from championship athletes to busy office workers.

Called the "Big 3," they are "core stabilization exercises."

1. Bird Dog
2. Side Plank
3. Curl Up

One review in *Frontiers in Public Health* compared 20 different forms of exercise to see which improved back health the most. The good news was that doing any exercise at all beat doing nothing, but core stabilization exercises came out on top.

McGill said, "The Big 3 came from experimentation converging on the very best exercises to address the mechanisms of pain." These exercises work by enhancing your core's stiffness so it can support loads and "eliminate the micromovements that cause pain."

At a minimum, I'd suggest doing a single set of each exercise a couple of times a week, but a more frequent and consistent routine will provide the best results.

- **Bird Dog:** Hold your opposite arm and leg stretched out for 10 seconds. That's 1 rep. Do 5 to 10 reps on each side.
- **Side Plank:** Hold the top position for 5 to 10 seconds. That's 1 rep. Do 5 to 10 reps on each side.
- **Curl Up:** Hold the top position for 5 to 10 seconds. That's 1 rep. Do 5 to 10 reps, then change which knee is "up" and repeat.

You can find a detailed video of each of these exercises to help with proper form and execution by scanning the following QR code:

## AVOID THE MOST COMMON WALKING-WITH-WEIGHT INJURY

In 2004, the United States was in a full-on war in Iraq and Afghanistan. We had troops on the ground—especially Special Operations troops, for whom rucking is the foundation of combat and fitness.

With that in mind, a group of US Army researchers decided to go deep down the rabbit hole of research on walking with weight. They looked at everything. The resultant report is hundreds of pages, part of which investigates injuries.

The scientists found that foot blisters—those mild but totally annoying sores—are the most common rucking injury. For example, one study examined the injuries of 355 soldiers during a 12.5-mile max-effort march. In that study, blisters made up 38 percent of the injuries.

Another study analyzed 218 infantry soldiers during a 5-day, 100-mile march. In that case, blisters comprised 48 percent of the injuries compared to foot pain's 19 percent.

You may not consider blisters a "real" injury, but the military does. For example, Napoleon lost one of his most critical battles because his troops didn't practice proper foot care. The scientists wrote:

> *Blisters can cause extreme discomfort, prevent service members from completing marches, and lead to many days of limited activity. If they are not properly managed, especially in field conditions, they can progress to more serious problems.*

I think we all know how blisters happen. But just in case you need clarity, here's how the army researchers described it: "Blisters result from friction between the socks and skin, a product of point pressures exerted by the boot and the foot."

More importantly, here are six ways you can protect your feet from blisters:

### 1. Toughen your feet

A 1995 army study found "sudden increases in march intensity or distance will probably make blisters more likely, regardless of training regularity." The researchers' takeaway was that your feet need time to adapt and "toughen." And that takes putting in miles but not doing too much too soon.

**Your move:** Walk with weight regularly. If you start to get a hot spot, stop immediately. Repeat a couple days later. That'll push the boundaries of what your feet are capable of over time and make blisters less likely to form.

## 2. Get shoes that fit

The US Army Public Health Center explained that good-fitting shoes are critical. They recommended:

- You should have about ½ inch from your big toe to the shoe's end.
- The shoes should be wide enough but not loose around your heel.
- You should lace your shoes snugly but not too tightly.

One simple trick that often fixes hot spots is to loosen or tighten your shoes.

## 3. Keep your feet dry

The scientists discovered that moisture increases the frictional forces against your skin, increasing the likelihood of getting a blister. Obviously, it can be challenging to keep your feet perfectly dry because feet sweat.

To control sweat, you can apply antiperspirant to your feet. Some anecdotal reports and case studies suggest this works, although the research is inconclusive. You can also try wearing merino wool or synthetic fiber socks. These fabrics push moisture away from your feet. They're also more durable, and merino will stay warm when wet.

## 4. Bring extra socks on a long walk

"There is one item of (military) gear that can be the difference between a live grunt and a dead grunt: socks." Those are the wise words of Lieutenant Dan from the movie *Forrest Gump*.

He's not wrong. If your feet become moist and you feel a hot spot, switch out your socks.

## 5. Treat a hot spot immediately

Most of us aren't walking with weight because we're on a military mission (to those of you who are, thanks for your service). We're usually walking rather close to home for general fitness. In these cases, just head home as soon as you feel a blister coming on and give your feet time to heal.

If you're out on a long walk or backpacking trip and get a hot spot, however, treat it immediately. Try any of the following:

- Switch out your socks.
- Adjust your shoes (loosen or tighten the laces).
- Use a moleskin or duct tape patch to cover the area.

These tips will prevent a hot spot from getting worse and will make your life (and your walk!) less miserable.

## 6. Go lighter

The likelihood of getting a blister rises with how much weight you have on your back because more weight puts more pressure on your skin and leads your foot to move more inside your shoe (due to pushing off and braking harder).

One way to lessen the rubbing on a hot spot is to temporarily lighten the load. Another way is to change how you carry the load. For example, carry the pack at your front for a while, which will alter how your foot moves in your shoe.

### How to treat a blister

The military researchers laid out what to do if a hot spot lapses into a blister.

- If the blister is intact: Drain it, leave the top in place, and put a light cover on it.
- If the blister is torn: Remove the top, place some antibiotic ointment on it, and put a bandage on it.

Should be simple! Of course, to be safe, it is recommended that you see a doctor for any serious injuries.

# 8

# PACKS, VESTS, AND GEAR

The question I get asked most often is some variation of "Should I use a backpack or a weighted vest?" It's a great question. Over the years, I've seen more people out in my neighborhood carrying weight in packs and vests. It's a beautiful thing.

When you're just getting started and considering buying gear, however, it can be hard to figure out which to use. As you may have guessed, I've done the research here, and my big takeaway for you is this: *That* you carry weight is far more important than *how* you carry it. Use whatever method you enjoy most and will use most often. When it comes to exercise, consistency is more important than nitty-gritty details.

In this chapter, I'll cover the most popular gear options and explain the pros and cons of each. This may help guide your choice.

## A BACKPACK YOU ALREADY HAVE AT HOME

**Upside:** It's free and immediately available. It allows you to start right now.
**Downside:** Because the bag isn't designed to carry weight for the sake of it, it takes a lot more effort to get the weight to sit comfortably in the pack. You may have to use odd objects for weight and jury-rig the weight to sit higher and tighter to your back. That said, having to do that is not the end of the world.

**Note:** I see using packs and weights you have at home as a great on-ramp. You can use what you have available to get started and make sure you like weighted walking, then you can upgrade your equipment.

## A HIKING BACKPACK

**Upside:** Hiking backpacks have more structure and are better designed to carry weight than the average bookbag, and many people already have one. They have ideal features like a hip belt or sternum strap and dedicated pockets for water, snacks, and a jacket.
**Downside:** Hiking backpacks have the same issues as regular backpacks—you'll still have to use odd objects as weight and do a lot of work to get the weight to sit right. Some people may also not want to look like they're headed out for a hike when they're just walking around their neighborhood.

**Note:** If you want a hiking backpack brand that can carry heavier weight and double as a great pack for outdoor pursuits, look to brands like Eberlestock and Mystery Ranch. Their packs are designed for hunters who often must pack out heavy loads of meat. Some even have sleeves that can hold a steel plate. That makes them more than able to carry any weights you'd walk with.

## GORUCK GEAR

**Upside:** Indestructible—this brand's gear lasts forever. Some models, like the Rucker 4.0, have sleeves in the main compartment that hold heavy weight plates tight to your upper back. They also offer various rucking-specific packs and vests.
**Downside:** Expensive. A setup costs anywhere from $300 to $400. Accessories like a hip belt and a weight plate cost extra. The products are based on military packs and can sometimes fit poorly, especially for women and people with smaller frames, leading to issues like sores. The bags also have a military look. Some people like that, but others prefer to avoid it.

## PLATE CARRIER WEIGHT VESTS

**Upside:** These vests are well-built and mimic bulletproof vests, which makes them ideal for first responders.
**Downside:** These vests are based on body armor plate carriers worn by soldiers and law enforcement. They're

designed to stop bullets, not to walk efficiently. The front plate can sit heavily on your chest. Many people find that the design makes it harder to breathe and leads to overheating. The design also makes it nearly impossible for some women to wear due to their breasts.

The weights are large steel plates, which means adjustments are typically made in 10-pound increments. If you load the front and back of the vest with the lightest plates you can find, it often still ends up being 20 pounds, which may be too heavy for some. Plates from brands other than the vest's manufacturer sometimes won't fit.

**Note:** Popular brands that make plate carrier weight vests are 5.11 Tactical, GORUCK, and Rogue.

## HYPERWEAR VEST

**Upside:** This vest is much more pliable than military-style vests. The weight is embedded within the vest as tiny steel beads that run throughout the vest in pockets. You can also adjust the weight in smaller increments.

**Downside:** The vest zips up the front, which can make it harder for women with larger breasts to wear. The design looks similar to a bullet-proof vest. It fully covers the chest, with weight on your rib cage. The vests aren't available with more than 20 pounds of weight. Lots of excess cordage hangs from them.

## WALKFULLY

**Upside:** No military vibe; beautifully designed. The designs better accommodate the female body. No weight is placed on the chest in any of the products, including vests, which improves breathing mechanics and heat disbursement.

The brand offers a pack, a vest that doesn't cover your chest, and two hip packs, which put the weight at your hips. The weights start at approachable levels and allow you to add more weight as you improve your fitness. For example, the vest weight ranges from 12 to 24 pounds, and the pack starts at 14 pounds but can go up to 50 pounds.

**Downside:** The pack maxes out at 50 pounds. It isn't built for people who want to walk with more than 50 pounds. People who really want to push the weight may want to look to another brand.

**Note:** Full transparency—I recently cofounded the Walkfully brand of gear, and in doing so, my partners and I hired a top pack designer to be sure the gear was both functional and comfortable. Our mission is simple: Inspire more people to walk with weight comfortably, joyfully, and inclusively.

If you are having trouble deciding which type of backpack or vest is right for you, feel free to message me on my Substack, *Two Percent* (twopct.com), about this topic. I'll happily point you to a product that I think will work best for you.

## What clothing to wear

It's best to wear a wool or synthetic top and avoid cotton. Cotton is 100 percent hydrophilic, meaning it retains moisture. When cotton gets wet, it holds water. It can cling to your skin, which impedes your body's ability to cool itself because sweat cools us by evaporating. If cotton gets wet from sweat in the cold, it has the opposite problem—it can lead you to get too cold and result in issues like hypothermia.

Wool and synthetic layers, on the other hand, pull moisture away from your body and lead it to evaporate faster, keeping you dryer—cooler in summer and warmer in winter. This is why your first layer should be thin and made of wool or synthetic fabric.

- Wool is generally warmer and manages body odor, but it's less durable, more expensive, and doesn't dry as quickly.
- Synthetic is generally cheaper, dries more quickly, and is more durable, but it can retain odor (I've found that odor retention is more of an issue in humid climates).

Of course, if you're just going for a short walk around your neighborhood, you'll be fine with cotton. But for longer walks in hot or cold weather, you probably want to go with wool or synthetic material.

On cold days, dress so you're a bit chilly when you start. Once you start moving, you'll warm up. If you overdress, you'll overheat and become sweaty or will have to stop to remove a layer.

If you live in a hot environment, select a weighted pack that doesn't cover your chest. For example, use a backpack, weight vest from WalkFully, or a weighted hip pack. These will allow air to flow over your chest as you sweat, keeping you cooler.

## PACKS VS. VESTS

Of course, both packs and vests have different benefits and downsides. As I mentioned earlier, I've done my own research on the topic of carrying weight in a pack versus a vest and spoken to various experts. But I wanted to pressure test my ideas, so I spoke to Kelly Starrett, a doctor of physical therapy. Kelly is considered one of the brightest public minds in human movement and physical activity. He's worked with professional teams in all major sports, helped Olympians win gold medals, and consults on physical preparedness for the military.

My research and conversation with Kelly led me to eight different scenarios in which I've determined whether walking with a pack or vest would be more beneficial.

### If you're covering long distances . . .

**WINNER: BACKPACKS**

Kelly made a great point right off the bat, 34 seconds into our conversation: "First, I need to point out that weight vests were never intended to carry weight," he said. "Weighted vests were originally designed to protect people if they got shot." Soldiers and law enforcement officers wear vests that weigh anywhere from 8 to 20 pounds to stop bullets.

When you look at how people around the world and throughout time have carried weight, you tend to see two approaches: on their head or on their back.

Let's quickly cover the first method: on your head. I don't think you're going to do that—and you probably shouldn't. But there is some fascinating research about it.

A study in the journal *Nature* found that women from the Kikuyu and Luo tribes in East Africa can carry up to 20 percent of their body weight on their head without burning any more calories than if they were walking with nothing. Those women have been carrying weight on their heads their entire lives, so their bodies are highly trained to be incredibly efficient at carrying weight that way.

But our goal when walking with weight for fitness is to burn extra calories.

This brings us to the second method: carrying weight on your back. Most people carry heavier loads on their backs. For example, I've seen people from Bhutan to Baghdad carrying everything from big bundles of wood to giant bags of fruit and vegetables on their backs.

I've never seen anyone instinctually distribute a heavy weight across their front and their back, like a vest does.

**The reason is simple:** Over long distances and with heavier loads, it's more efficient and safer to have more of the weight on your back.

This is because backpacks allow us to "lean" away from the weight (or into the front of the straps, depending on how you view it), and the physics work in our favor.

We can resist the weight using our abs and posterior muscles, which are generally strong because we're forward-driven creatures. And if those tire, we can default to using our skeletal system.

Kelly explained it like this: "With a backpack on, there's a force you can resist against that is straight up and down. If you put a heavy backpack on even a child, the child intuitively knows how to lean into it and stabilize."

But this intuition doesn't necessarily kick in when the weight is enveloping your body, like it does with a vest. You have nothing to resist against—to sort of lean into. This means your muscles must create all that stability.

When our muscles tire, we often begin to slump, and the weight of the vest consumes us, leading to poor walking mechanics.

Kelly said, "Let's say I put a 250-pound backpack on you. It would suck, but you'd be able to stand by leaning forward. But if I wrapped that same 250-pound weight around you in a weight vest, you'd probably collapse because you had nothing to lean into."

He continued: "This is why I think using a backpack is much more sustainable for relatively heavier loads and for longer periods of time. For example, think of thru-hikers who are hiking 20 miles a day. These people have the option of putting loads on their backs and fronts. But these people are all putting light loads on their backs because it allows them to hike faster and be the most efficient."

**The takeaway:** Vests and backpacks are equally good for loads up to around 10 to 15 percent of your body weight. But if you have more than 10 to 15 percent of your body weight and are planning to walk a far distance, you might want to use a backpack or vest that distributes more of the load onto your back.

## If you want something versatile . . .

**WINNER: BACKPACKS OR VESTS WITH AN OPEN CHEST AND POCKETS**

In 1996, two groups of scientists from the US Army convened to study walking with weight to understand how soldiers were impacted by backpacks versus vests. They found: "Backpacks appear to provide greater versatility. . . . The [vest] can inhibit movement . . . can be burdensome to put on and remove . . . [and] can also induce ventilatory impairment and greater heat stress symptoms."

That said, the study used rather heavy vests, and the same effect likely wouldn't happen with a vest that weighs around 10 to 15 percent of your body weight.

Still, the scientists found heavier vests were:

- Harder to move in because you also have weight in front of you.
- Harder to put on and take off.
- Harder to breathe in while wearing.
- More likely to lead you to overheat.

We'll cover more info on those final two points below.

**The takeaway:** Use a backpack or a lighter vest that doesn't cover your chest. With backpacks and light vests that include pockets, you can also pack snacks, a light jacket, and a water bottle. Most vests that cover your front don't let you do this.

## If you want to lessen your risk of injury . . .

**WINNER: BACKPACKS OR VESTS LESS THAN 15 PERCENT OF YOUR BODY WEIGHT**

In the laboratory, weight vests appear to cause the fewest changes to how you walk. Scientists in Hong Kong found that "[vest] loads resulted in a more upright walking posture and induced fewer postural deviations from normal walking."

But when you wear a pack, as we covered, you lean forward to resist the weight more. We don't usually walk leaning slightly forward, so the implication is that walking with a vest causes fewer perturbations in your gait, or walking style, and leads to fewer injuries.

This means it's quite possible that under controlled conditions, vests may have a lower risk of injury.

But life isn't a laboratory. In the study, participants walked only 10 minutes. This is when it becomes useful to look at real-world experience.

Kelly told me about his experience working with soldiers who wear body armor vests that can weigh up to 35 pounds. He explained: "People end up slumping in heavy body armor vests. We see it all the time when I work with the Marine Corps. When people get fatigued, the strategy is to lean forward to bend over at the waist. But when you're wearing a vest, there's nothing to lean against. You can't find equilibrium, so you default to rounding inside the vest, which we've seen time and time again cause issues."

The idea stems from what we learned in point number one: As you tire and lean forward, the front load pulls you further forward.

It's like an anchor rounding your back. Eventually, your lower back muscles can tire, putting that weight on your spine. And that can be bad news, especially if you're using heavier loads.

**The takeaway:** A pack will be best for loads above 10 to 15 percent of your body weight. Weight vests also work great as long as you don't go much over 10 to 15 percent of your body weight or use a vest where a greater proportion of the weight is at the back.

## If you want a stronger core and back . . .

### WINNER: BACKPACKS OR VESTS THAT DISTRIBUTE MORE LOAD TO YOUR BACK

In 1984, two biomechanists at the University of Waterloo measured how back muscles activate when people walk with weight in a backpack. They had a small group of men toss on a 42-pound backpack. Then they used an electromyography (EMG) machine to measure muscle activity.

The findings were counterintuitive. The scientists found that your low-back muscles—called the erector spinae—actually activated *less* when the people walked with a weighted pack compared with walking without weight. Another study found this rule held until people loaded their backpacks with over 66 to 88 pounds (read, probably not a weight I'd recommend).

But, clearly, walking with a weighted backpack is more physically demanding than walking without any weight. So, *something* had to make up for the lack of activation from the back muscles. The answer: Your abs pick up the slack.

The scientists explained that when you toss on a weighted backpack and lean slightly forward to counter the weight, it reduces the torque on your lower back but increases the tension on your abs. That ab work is a great thing for modern people. Most people who sit often at work and home have weak core muscles.

This may be why renowned back expert Stuart McGill, PhD, told me walking with a weighted pack can be excellent for back health. Reducing the torque on your low back and giving your spine some motion generally do good things for back problems.

He said: "The spine tends to like gentle motion. There's no such thing as a common treatment for everyone. However, on average, people's discs and spines enjoy a little bit of motion. . . . In our earlier studies, one of our recommended therapies for people recovering from posterior disc bulges was to put a load in their backpack and carry the load. Only 20 or 25 pounds placed low in the backpack and close to their back."

Not to mention, having a stronger core is associated with less risk of back injury. And it can help you perform better in everything from running to weightlifting, playing pickleball to chasing down your kids.

**The takeaway:** Backpacks or vests that put more of the load at your back tend to work your core harder and may make your back more resilient (assuming you don't overload yourself).

## If you want to breathe better and not overheat . . .

### WINNER: BACKPACKS OR VESTS THAT DON'T COVER YOUR CHEST

This seems rather obvious, but if you put a bunch of weight on your chest, it's going to make it harder to breathe.

Science is often about confirming the obvious, and when scientists analyzed the research, they noted that vests "can induce ventilatory impairments." That's jargon for "make it hard to breathe." This occurs in weight vests that place big weight plates across your back and chest. This doesn't happen with backpacks. It also doesn't happen with vests that are designed to leave your chest open.

One wise exercise physiologist, Ben Olliver, who is the chief performance officer at Supra Human, a fitness training company, put it quite eloquently when he told me, "I use a backpack instead of a weight vest because the vest just makes it hard as f*ck to breathe." Granted, he'd tried weight vests that slap the weight across your chest and likes to walk with rather heavy weights

Then there's heat. A vest that fully covers your chest is like wearing a steel insulation blanket. Because vests wrap the weight around your body, it's harder for you to dissipate heat. That might be a good thing in winter, but you can always layer up, and in summer you'll get uncomfortably hot.

**The takeaway:** A backpack opens your front, making it easier to breathe and allowing for sweating to do its job. Air can flow over the sweat on the front of your body, leading to evaporative cooling. This also happens with vests that leave your chest open, like the one made by WalkFully.

## If you're worried about loading the weight correctly . . .

**WINNER: VESTS**

As we covered earlier in the book, where you place the load is important when walking with weight. You want it tight to your body. This is easier to do with a vest because the weight is usually fixed in the vest. You can't really choose where to load the weight.

If you're using any old backpack and some random weights around the house, like dumbbells or books, it can be harder to fit and load the weight correctly. You must jury-rig the backpack so the load is tight.

If your pack is poorly loaded, with loose straps and weight hanging at the bottom, it might sway, and that swaying can create movement problems as you walk with weight.

One trainer told me, "Because of that nuance, it makes me say, okay, for most people, wear a vest. Vests are pretty much idiot-proof, as long as you can breathe in the thing, the weight is going to be distributed more or less correctly."

**The takeaway:** If you're using a vest, just strap the thing on. No thought necessary. Ideally, use one that leaves your chest open so you can breathe easily. If you're using a random pack from home and odd objects for weight, try to get the weight close to your back (rather than having it "flopping outward"). For example, place weight in the laptop sleeve.

## If you don't want to look like you're going into combat . . .

### WINNER: BACKPACKS OR A WEIGHT VEST THAT LEAVES YOUR CHEST OPEN

I had a friend in college who was incredibly lovable, but he seemed to have missed the day when the good Lord handed out IQ points.

One day, my friend decided to walk around campus wearing a weight vest. It was one that fully covered his front, the type sold by companies that make military-style gear. It also happened to be a cold and windy winter day in New England, so he put on a full knit face mask to stay warm. Picture a kid walking around a college campus in a full knit face mask and what appears to be a bulletproof vest. This set off some alarm bells—and my friend was immediately detained by campus police.

Weight vests that fully cover your front make you like you're wearing a bulletproof vest. It's not ideal to walk around your neighborhood appearing like you're preparing to throw a violent coup against the HOA.

**The takeaway:** Backpacks are far more normal to wear and see in public—we see them every day in schools, airports, and around the city. So are weight vests that leave your front open, like those we have at WalkFully. These mimic running vests, and we see these often on the runners in our neighborhoods and out on the trails.

## If you want to do workouts while wearing it . . .

**WINNER: VESTS**

Body weight workouts—think push-ups, squats, lunges, step-ups—are a fantastic way to build your strength, boost your cardio, and improve your mobility. Adding a bit of weight makes them even more effective.

Vests are the winner here. They hug you and distribute the weight evenly around your torso. This allows for a full range of motion with minimal interference.

Backpacks, on the other hand, bounce and shift around more, which can make the movements awkward. The pack can slide around your back and bang you up.

**The takeaway:** With vests, the weight becomes part of you, not an extension of you that you have to manage. That makes them ideal for body weight workouts.

## If you want to scale the weight as your fitness improves . . .

**WINNER: BACKPACKS OR EASILY ADJUSTABLE VESTS**

Vests are typically limited to lower weights—most cap out around 20 pounds.

Amazon sells vests that go up to 150 pounds, but they tend to be bulky, rigid, and awkward. Not to mention, adjusting the load is a hassle, and it's nearly impossible to use a significantly lighter load with them.

Backpacks make it far easier to use a range of weights. You can toss in 5 pounds or 75 pounds with relative ease.

**The takeaway:** Backpacks are a better option for those who frequently change weights (I use a range from 20 to 50 pounds (or heavier, if I have a specific event I'm preparing for). Some vests, like those from WalkFully, also make it easy to quickly adjust the weight.

## If you're a military member or law enforcement officer . . .

**WINNER: MILITARY-STYLE VESTS**

Military and law enforcement groups must wear vests at work for safety. They often have to sprint, jog, or fight in those heavy vests. So, for those groups, it makes sense to train in military-style vests to better prepare for the real thing. If you're a military or law enforcement officer, thanks for your service and know that a mix of exercise using a backpack and a vest seems like a great idea.

*We've just gone a bit down the rabbit hole of packs versus vests.* Your brain might be reeling. So, I'll go back to my initial message: It is far more important that you walk with weight than what you carry it in. Figure out what works best for you and lean in. I will say, however, that most people find a backpack or vest that keeps their chest open the best option for walking with weight.

Part Three

# LIVE THE PRACTICE

# 9

# ADOPT A TWO PERCENT MINDSET

My *Two Percent* Substack newsletter goes out three times a week to hundreds of thousands of people across 204 countries. Its name comes from a study that discovered only 2 percent of people take the stairs when there's an escalator available.

To me, however, that figure isn't *really* about the stairs. It's a metaphor for our current health crisis and how to live better. We often avoid the easiest wins, and it's killing us. Inactivity is a main contributor to the 10 leading causes of death. Yet 98 percent of us avoid the simple, obvious, healthy choice of taking the stairs.

The figure is about becoming one of the rare breed of humans who choose the slightly harder path that delivers giant dividends over the long term. Research shows that the 2 percent of people who consistently take the stairs—and apply that Two Percent mindset to other areas of life—live longer, better, more impactful lives.

One of the simplest ways you can enhance your body, mind, and spirit is to adopt the Two Percent mindset—to say yes to the little opportunities we have to do the slightly harder thing that gives us a massive long-term reward.

We can apply the mindset to walking with weight, and this chapter covers a handful of clever ways to do just that.

## TAKE CALLS WHILE WALKING WITH WEIGHT

During the pandemic, incessant phone and video conferences were making me lazy and crazy. My steps were down, as was my mental health. One day, I had yet another work call—it was my fifth of the day—and I decided to do something different: I tossed on a light pack and took my work call while walking throughout my neighborhood.

Walking with a pack not only helped me sneak in a ton of activity when I would have been just sitting at my desk, but it also changed the meeting's dynamics. I was more focused, with fewer digital distractions—no looking at emails or scrolling the internet during the meeting. I was also more energized and happier afterward.

The numbers don't lie.

- People who took walking meetings increased their scores on standardized productivity and creativity tests by 8 percent and 60 percent, respectively.
- The average meeting lasts 54 minutes, so you'll log about 6,000 steps. That number of steps drops your risk of death by 40 to 50 percent compared with walking just 3,500 steps a day. (And that's only from one meeting . . . walking meetings help you get far more steps across a day.)
- You'll also supercharge each of those steps. When you factor in the extra calories burned from walking with the pack, you'll use up at least 20 percent more calories per step.

I've been walking with a light pack on my back during meetings when possible ever since. But it hasn't always been perfect—and I've had to solve some problems along the way. Here are my six key strategies to make your walking meetings a success.

## 1. Scout your route

In one of my very first rucking meetings, I was walking down the sidewalk when the call garbled, leading me to scream "CAN YOU HEAR ME?" a few times. Then the call dropped. I had to frantically redial into the conference line, apologize, and ask to be filled in on what I missed. It was frustrating for all involved—and a bad look!

The world is full of vortexes where full bars of cell phone service seemingly evaporate for no good reason.

**The solution:** Before your first walking meeting, stroll your planned route. Call your mom or grandma along the way—she'd love to hear from you—to ensure the route has reliable service throughout.

## 2. Use less weight

Walking with weight during meetings is a sneaky and effective way to get fit. A few months after I started, I found myself leaner and with better endurance. So, I thought more would equal more—I increased the weight and speed. This was a miscalculation. I forgot that I was walking during a meeting, not taking a meeting during a workout.

If you overload your pack and walk too fast, you'll end up sweating and breathing heavily, which distracts you from the meeting (and is also rather awkward for others on the line).

**The solution:** Lighten your pack by roughly half.

- If you normally walk with 30 pounds, drop the weight to 15 or 20.
- If you walk with 50, drop the weight to 30.
- If you normally walk with 20, try 10.
- Or just leave the weighted pack at home and walk. Anything is better than sitting.

**A guideline:** If you can't speak clearly throughout your walk, including walking up hills, your weight is too heavy. You'll still see a massive benefit from any weight you use. Again, moving beats sitting.

## 3. Favor nature

In previous chapters, we learned that the average American spends 93 percent of their time indoors. Our modern removal from the outdoors is linked to the epidemic of mental and physical health issues sweeping the country. Any time outside is good. But remember, walking through a paved-over parking lot versus on a tree-lined path impacts us differently.

**The solution:** If possible, favor more natural areas during your walking meeting. Find a park, trail, or tree-lined street.

Spending just 20 minutes a few times a week in natural spaces—the kind you can find in a city park or street flanked by a lot of green—decreases stress and increases productivity and health markers.

## 4. Find a quieter route

I thought I was set once I discovered a good route that got service and moved through some nature. I was wrong.

One day, a park I walked through was packed with children who were all screaming as they played tag. Another day, a house along my route had landscapers working with blaring leaf blowers. Garbage trucks were another big noise polluter. These all impacted my ability to hear and speak on the call.

**The solution:** Seek a silent route and stay alert for unexpected noises. As you walk, look for noise land mines. For example, garbage trucks, workers, lawn mowers, or leaf blowers. Also use your phone's mute button liberally and consider noise-canceling headphones.

And, to be fair to the outdoors, unexpected noise happens indoors all the time. Think barking dogs, doorbell rings, and yelling kids.

## 5. Bring coworkers

Cheryl from accounting and Eric from HR aren't actually awkward and personality-less. What's awkward is trying to have a real conversation with Cheryl and Eric while you're crammed into some drop-ceiling, fluorescently lit, windowless room. Most office conference rooms are where personalities go to die.

The good news: People come out of their shell once you get them outside and moving.

One study in the *Journal of Occupational and Environmental Medicine* found that in-person walking meetings improved communication and camaraderie among coworkers compared with sit-down office meetings.

**The solution:** If you work in person, ask your colleagues if they'd like to walk during the meeting. Sell it—tell them about all the benefits. The research suggests that together, walking shoulder to shoulder, you'll be more productive, come to better solutions, and enjoy the meeting.

## 6. Walk to healthy places

Having a fun destination to walk to can motivate you and your coworkers to do more walking meetings. But researchers at the University of South Florida found that many people who did walking meetings walked to a donut shop for an extra-long maple bar or to Starbucks for an extra-large Frappuccino with whipped cream.

The scientists agreed that it's fine to do that sometimes. One upside of walking rather than sitting is that it gives you more room for fried, frosting-glazed indulgences. But the scientists worried that having too many walking meetings that end in hundreds of calories of sugar, salt, and fat may backfire.

**The solution:** A coffee shop or café gives your meeting a destination and a reward at the end, incentivizing more participation. But once you're there, get something calorie-free, for example, a black coffee or cold brew.

## WALK AIRPORT TERMINALS WHILE WAITING FOR FLIGHTS

When I was promoting my last book, *Scarcity Brain*, I traveled to about four states a week. My life became an act of moving from airplane to hotel to interview—rinse and repeat.

Travel often kills our health and fitness. We sit and eat too much and skip workouts. But during my three-month book tour, I was able to stay fit. I didn't gain weight, and I felt far better throughout my travels than usual. The reason: I spent a lot of time walking around airports while wearing my pack.

If I had a 2-hour layover, I'd walk with my carry-on backpack for about 1 hour and 30 minutes. In that time, I'd log 4 to 5 miles of walking.

If I had to wait 40 minutes to board (yes, I'm one of those people who arrive at airports early), I'd walk around and cover more than 2 miles. Sometimes I'd listen to music or a podcast. Other times I'd people-watch.

I could have sat in some uncomfortable terminal chair and buried my head in my phone like everyone else. But I knew I was going to be sitting on a plane for hours. So why sit more? Why not take the opportunity to get in some life-enhancing movement?

I also learned a few valuable lessons. These four tips will help you, too.

PS, I've applied them to waiting for flights, but you can get creative and use them any time you have a wait—whether you have a pack or not.

### 1. Don't worry about the weight

The point of walking through an airport carrying weight isn't to walk with weight just like you would in a dedicated workout. We're not trying to hammer through the terminal like we're training for Navy SEAL selection camp. Rather, the point is to sneak in light exercise instead of sitting. The normal weight of your carry-on is fine.

My pack usually contains:

- A couple books and a Kindle.
- A liter of water.
- Snacks like apples and jerky sticks.
- A computer, a bunch of cords, and maybe a camera.
- Clothes and toiletries if it's a quick trip.

Total weight: 15 to 20 pounds. This is less than the weight I usually use at home. But that's okay!

### 2. Get creative with how you carry

I usually travel with a single pack. But if a trip is more than 72 hours—or if it's one where I need better clothes than just

T-shirts and jeans—I'll usually keep my clothes and toiletries in a duffel bag. I always carry on my luggage because:

- Waiting for your luggage at the baggage claim sucks.
- Luggage gets lost all the time (AMA the time my checked bag full of safety gear got lost during a semi-dangerous trip to report on the drug trade in Iraq).
- Carrying-on means I get to carry another bag through the airport—i.e., more weight to walk with.

Duffel bags allow you to sneak in even more work because you must carry them. They also fit into the overhead bins better than roller bags because they're more pliable. You can literally just shove them in crevices between roller bags.

My advice for carrying a duffel in addition to your backpack: Switch how you carry the duffel as you walk.

- Hold it in your left hand for a while.
- Then hold it in your right hand.
- Then sling it over your right shoulder, then your left shoulder.

Remember, carrying weight at one side works your core harder than perfectly balancing the load between sides or on your back. That offset load can enhance your performance and improve your back health and movement quality.

### 3. Don't sweat it

I often post dumb videos of myself walking through airports wearing my backpack on social media. People sometimes respond by telling me they can't walk in an airport because they're worried about boarding the plane soaking in sweat.

I get it. I don't want to board a plane sweaty, either. People all sweat differently—some sweat more than others, and there are a variety of reasons for that.

To avoid sweating while you stroll the terminals, you can do a few things:

- **Don't go too hard.** Again, we're not training for the Olympics here. Walk at whatever pace you're comfortable with. Slow down if you start to sweat and don't want to. Again, it beats sitting.
- **Get an iced drink.** Another way to stay cool: Buy a drink with ice, like a water or fountain Diet Coke, and sip the drink and chew on its ice as you walk. Doing that can reduce your core temperature and the likelihood that you'll sweat.
- **Change your shirt.** If you know you might sweat and still want to walk the airport, carry an extra T-shirt in your pack. Change into it before you get on the plane.
- **Get lounge access.** A couple of years ago, I upgraded my credit card to one that gets me into lounges. I think these cards only make financial sense if you travel frequently (and know how to leverage the perks to offset the stupid-high annual fees). The upside is that many (but not all) lounges have showers. This means you could walk the airport hard and fast—like you're training for the Olympics—then take a shower and change your clothes before your flight. I did this in the Seoul, South Korea, airport to offset 24 hours of sitting on planes.
- **Improve your cardio.** This is a long-term solution. Generally, unfit people will start sweating sooner and at lower exercise intensities than will fit people. So, walk

with weight more often at home, and you'll soon find you're able to avoid sweating as you walk terminals.

### 4. Calculate your distance, if you care

If you want a general sense of how far you've walked, do the following:

- Start a timer on your watch. Walk. Stop the timer when you're finished. Take your total minutes and divide it by 20. That's roughly the number of miles you walk. Generally, 20 minutes of walking is about equal to 1 mile at an average walking pace.
- Or, if your phone has a step counter, look at your steps before you start. Then look at them after. Two thousand steps is about 1 mile of walking.

## DO CHORES WITH WEIGHT ON YOUR BACK

When I surveyed readers of *Two Percent* about their favorite tips to walk with weight better, many lauded the benefits of wearing their packs at home. Here are a few things people wrote:

> *Wearing my pack with smaller weights while I do everyday chores (mowing the lawn, etc.) helped get me used to moving with the weight and more comfortable with walking with weight and walking farther distances.*
>
> **—Don, 71**

> *Wear your pack when you vacuum! It's so helpful. It really got me used to the weight and allowed me to walk farther distances.*
>
> **—Leah, 36**

> *When I was just starting, I did yard work while wearing a 20-pound weighted pack. It made cutting the lawn a lot more challenging and built me a good base of fitness. Because I was at home, I could take off the weight at any time if I felt tired. I still do this even though I'm now a much stronger rucker.*
>
> —**Mary, 49**

These accounts all track with me. For example, I recently did a 45-day hike—walking 20 to 30 miles a day with a pack on my back. To prepare for that, I'd load a pack with up to 45 pounds and do all sorts of chores around the house.

I'd clean, organize, work at my desk, vacuum, and more—all while loaded down like a military grunt. Sure, it was a little wacky. But I had only my dogs and wife there to make fun of me, which generally happens no matter what I do.

Here's why it was so useful: On a regular walk, we typically carry the weight for perhaps an hour and walk straight forward the entire time. But having the load on my back during chores meant that I:

1. Got more time with the weight on my back. That increased my fitness and prepared me to carry my pack for longer periods.
2. Was loaded down as I moved forward, backward, side to side, crouched, stood stationary, and more. That prepared me to exist with the load on my back on my hike, where I had to do all sorts of odd movements while wearing it.

Try it. Next time you have chores around the house, toss on your pack and go for it. You can always take it off when you get tired.

## USE A BABY CARRIER RATHER THAN A STROLLER

As we learned in chapter 2, backpacks were invented by clever mothers eons ago to carry children. Backpacks and slings are still useful devices for carrying kids today. And it turns out that our kids may get far more developmental benefits when they're carried compared with being in a stroller.

A team of international scientists recently analyzed the evolution of carrying our children and published their results in the journal *Infant Behavior and Development*. Here are some of the benefits they discovered:

### Kids learn language and human interaction better

When early humans started carrying their kids, it "opened up new ways of learning by observing visual and auditory stimuli simultaneously," the scientists wrote. Think about it. When you carry a child, they are in the middle of whatever you're doing, seeing and hearing the world as you do. The position "provide[s] a safe place and vantage point for learning in the most critical first year of life."

Perhaps most important is that the child is thrust into the middle of your interactions with other humans. They can watch other people's faces and mannerisms and eventually mirror their behaviors. It's how we begin to learn how to be a human with other humans.

### Kids gain important physical skills when carried

When you put an infant in a crib or car seat or lay them on the floor, they just sort of lay there. They are so weak they can hardly do anything but move their arms and legs a bit. But when you carry the child, some important physical skills are tested and developed.

1. **Head and neck control.** The infant must work their neck to keep their head upright. The researchers say this builds their vestibular system. That system is responsible for balance, knowing where their body is in space, and coordinating their movement with balance. It also begins to strengthen their core and stabilize muscles.
2. **Grip.** When you place your finger in a baby's hand, they'll grasp it. This is an innate reflex that likely evolved to help babies be carried. Babies reflexively grasp your skin or clothing when carried. The scientists wrote that this helps them stabilize their torso and triggers other bodily responses. It "keeps the infant a reflexively active participant while eliciting compensatory responses." Translation: They're learning how to move and react to the world.
3. **The "Moro reflex."** The Moro reflex is a response that kicks on when an infant loses balance. They extend their arms and legs, then pull their arms in, and sometimes cry. It's also been described as the "embracing reflex." Scientists think that its role is to teach an infant to cling to their parent and regain hold. It seems to help the baby's central nervous system develop. By carrying your infant, you're helping them build that reflex, develop body awareness, and enhance their physical development.
4. **Stepping.** When a baby touches their foot to a flat surface, they will make walking motions even though they are months from walking. This is elicited in carrying as well. Scientists think it helps babies cling

and adjust themselves when being carried, and it sets the movement patterns needed to eventually walk.

## Kids relax when carried

When a baby's mother picks them up, it's like they've both just popped a sedative. Both the mother's and baby's heart rates drop and sync up. Scientists call this the "transport response." The baby relaxes. Their stress markers drop, and they're likely to stop crying. Even when an infant isn't crying, being picked up and carried by their mom drops their heart rate (suggesting reduced stress).

- **Why this happens:** The scientists think the "transport response" improved survival. Let's say there's a predator nearby. If you pick up the baby and hug them tight and the baby stops crying or is less likely to cry, you'll be less likely to be detected.
- **One fascinating fact:** Heart rate doesn't drop as much if a stranger picks up the baby.
- **Most important:** The scientists wrote that babies who are frequently carried "appear more likely to thrive, becoming healthy and stable adults, even if their life is stressful. If infants do not receive the necessary body contact . . . the lack of it may cause long-term negative effects on their physical and mental health."

## Kids and parents become happier from carrying

Carrying not only seems to improve the happiness of babies, it also makes parents happier. For example, one study discovered that mothers who didn't have skin-to-skin contact with their kids experienced more symptoms of depression than did a group who carried their children every day. This holds for fathers, too.

## Of course, parents work their bodies when carrying kids

Babies need to be carried all the time until they are about 2 years old. Even then, you'll occasionally carry them.

Babies weigh an average of 7 to 8 pounds. They gain a pound or two a month until they reach age 2. The average 2-year-old weighs about 25 pounds. All that weight-carrying makes every movement more challenging—you're basically living life while carrying a dumbbell in your arms, at your side, slung across your front or back.

And because we carry kids in all different positions—hugged, in our right arm or left arm, at our right hip or left hip—and squirming around, it stimulates and strengthens all sorts of muscle groups, especially our core.

*Now that you know how to easily weave weighted walking into* your life to get more benefits, let's look at the harder path. In the next chapter, we'll cover five weighted walking challenges.

# 10

# CHALLENGE YOURSELF

Militaries around the world adopted packs and other carrying devices to haul gear into battle. Even prehistoric cave art depicts warriors heading into battles carrying gear. Ever since, militaries worldwide and throughout history have used walking with weight as their primary form of physical training.

While researching this book, I dug into old military data to understand how militaries throughout history have tested their soldiers, and I found a handful of fascinating rucking tests going back thousands of years.

**Big Warning:** I'm not suggesting anyone do these challenges as prescribed. As you'll soon see, they're tough. Really tough. These rucking challenges were designed to take soldiers to the edge of their endurance so they could march when their lives (and, sometimes, the fate of the world) depended on it.

I don't recommend trying these military challenges for

the average person, so here's what we'll do instead: I'll show you exactly how and why the military—whether it be the ancient Romans or the 10th Mountain Division—prescribed it. Then we'll adapt it so anyone can do it. Each challenge shows:

- The distance the soldiers would have to walk.
- The weight they'd have to walk with.
- The standard (usually a timeframe) they'd have to finish the walk in.
- How you can pare it down to better fit your own goals and abilities.

## I. THE ROMAN LEGIONNAIRES CHALLENGE

**Distance:** 22 miles
**Weight:** 45 pounds
**Standard:** Finish in 7 hours 20 minutes

The Roman Empire became one of the greatest in the world—expanding across Europe, North Africa, and Western Asia—thanks to the fitness of its soldiers. In 1921, military historian S. E. Stout wrote of Roman training: "The greatest advance in warfare in that time was in tactics, in the methods of organizing and ordering bodies of men so that they could be directed and maneuvered more effectively."

In other words, the military units that could quickly and tightly move themselves and their heavy gear from point A to point B—and still have enough energy to fight face-to-face—won wars.

To train, Roman soldiers loaded 45 pounds into their

rucksacks and marched on dirt roads throughout the empire. They'd cover 22 miles at a speed of about 3 miles an hour, which means the challenge took about 7 hours 20 minutes.

A funny aside: Roman "recruiters" preferred to draw soldiers from the country, not cities. Vegetius, a great military tactician of the time, said:

> *The youth of the country is better adapted to arms, for it is reared under the open sky and occupied in labor; it is trained to endure the sun and to spurn the shade; it knows nothing of baths nor of delicacies; it is simple-hearted and satisfied with little; its limbs are hardened to endure all kinds of toil; and it has grown accustomed in the country to handling implements.*

In other words, country people who did physical work outdoors were tougher than city people. Perhaps this challenge will help you become "hardened to endure all kinds of toil" as well.

## How to apply it

Walking for 7 hours 20 minutes across a single day is a remarkable and challenging way to get yourself outdoors for an extended period of time. Consider doing it once in your life or even annually. If that seems like a stretch, cut the time in half—walk 3 hours 40 minutes. And, no, you don't have to use 45 pounds of weight. Use a weight you're comfortable with or no weight at all.

If it feels challenging, remember that humans in the past used to spend most of the day on their feet, walking the earth.

Your ancestors had challenges such as this all the time—and you're surely capable of doing some variation of it.

## 2. CROMWELL READINESS RUCK

**Distance:** 15 miles
**Weight:** 35 pounds
**Standard:** Ability to finish at any time

Oliver Cromwell was a British politician and military leader who came to power in the 1600s. He led savage military campaigns across the United Kingdom. Churchill called him a military dictator, while others like John Milton and Thomas Carlyle called him a hero.

To understand just how loathed this guy was, consider this: Cromwell died of illness. In a power shift after his death, his enemies dug up his body and chopped off his head. Then, they displayed his head on a spike outside the Tower of London for 30 years.

His military prowess lay in his vicious tactics and insistence on having a fighting force that was prepared to move and strike at any moment. He required his soldiers to be able to march 15 miles with 35 pounds any time he asked them. If they couldn't finish the march, he wouldn't pay them.

### How to apply it

Cromwell's Challenge is an excellent test for the average person.

Depending on your weight, you may not use 35 pounds, but most relatively fit humans should be able to walk for 15 miles straight on a whim (even if it takes a while).

## 3. THE GERMAN ON-RAMP

**Distance:** Up to 12.5 miles
**Weight:** 57 pounds
**Standard:** Slowly work your way up to 12.5 miles

In the run-up to World War I, the German army needed to recruit and train as many soldiers as possible. But soldiers at the time weren't coming in as fit as they had in the past. The Industrial Revolution had led the average German to be less physically active.

German military leaders needed to bring their soldiers up to fighting fitness, so they built an on-ramp program. They'd load their soldiers with about 57 pounds, then they'd have them march 10 kilometers (or about 6 miles). From there, they'd add 1 kilometer to the march each week until the soldiers could march 20 kilometers, or about 12.5 miles.

### How to apply it

Don't use 57 pounds. That's *a lot* of weight. But there's deep wisdom in adding a kilometer to your walks each week when you're trying to build mileage. Consider running injuries. Research suggests that running too many miles too soon is the main cause of running injury. Our bodies get overwhelmed before they can adapt.

In my own life running and walking with weight, I've stayed injury-free by adding just half a mile (or roughly 1 kilometer) to my longer walks and runs each week if I'm trying to increase my distance.

You can do the same. Pick a starting distance and a goal distance for a long walk. For example, 3 miles to start and 7 miles as a goal. Week one, walk 3 miles. Each week from there, add about a half mile to your walk until you end up at 7 miles.

## 4. THE LION MARCH

**Distance:** 140 miles
**Weight:** 75 pounds
**Standard:** Finish once, go to war

The Chindits—Burmese for lions—were British special operations units that fought the Japanese in Burma in World War II. Roughly 3,000 of them rucked deep into Burma on Operation Longcloth. Their goal was to destroy railway and communications lines. One historian explained what they did like this: "They were loaded with huge 75-pound packs and marched unmercifully through man-killing terrain."

Major General Orde Charles Wingate, their leader, knew his troops would be marching long distances through some of the most savage jungle on earth. He required intense and long training, capped off by a final challenge before deployment. The final challenge: a 140-mile road march.

### How to apply it

It's smart to work up to a big "test" leading to an event to ensure you're physically ready. The military has done this for years to ensure that its soldiers are physically prepared.

Consider your own life and goals. What's a physical test you can create to ensure you're in peak shape? For example, I know my cardio is solid, and my legs are strong if I can load 45 pounds into a pack and walk briskly up a punishingly steep mountain near my house without stopping. The hike is about

4.5 miles and gains about 3,500 feet of elevation, ending at 11,000 feet above sea level.

You might consider working up to a certain goal distance to ensure you're ready for a big backpacking trip or vacation that involves a lot of walking.

## 5. 10TH MOUNTAIN DIVISION QUARTERLY

**Distance:** 25 miles
**Weight:** 94 pounds
**Standard:** Complete quarterly

The 10th Mountain Division began during World War II to conduct mountain warfare. Its members had to be fitter than most soldiers since they needed to climb at high altitude, cover jagged and snowy ground, and even ski—all while carrying packs loaded with gear that allowed them to fight and survive in extreme conditions.

This is why, every 3 months, the division would load their packs with their issued gear and cover 25 miles at a fast clip. It's important to note that their gear was heavier than most other military gear; their clothes were more insulated, and the unit also carried weather-resistant tents, stoves, skis, and more.

One study said they held an 11-minute/mile pace, but I think that's probably incorrect. Still, we can assume they were moving fast. In addition to the quarterly test, the division conducted a 100-mile march in 5 days once a year.

### How to apply it

A series of days of long walks is a great idea—even better if you can do them in the mountains. Go backpacking. Toss what you need to survive in a backpack and hit the mountains for a few days. Or you could just decide that one weekend every quarter you're going to do a super-long walk on both Saturday and Sunday.

Every year, I spend at least 3 days in the backcountry on a dedicated backpacking trip. It's one of my favorite things I do each year. It not only packs in a ton of walking with weight, but, as research shows, that extended time in wild nature is great for physical, mental, and spiritual health.

# 11

# TRAINING PLANS

This chapter covers several training plans that can improve your body, mind, and spirit through walking with weight, no matter your fitness level. They'll give you guidance on how to schedule a week of workouts based on your background and the time you have.

You'll find three plans that can be adapted to our ever-changing lifestyles. There's a time-crunched plan, moderate plan, and go-getter plan.

- Each plan is broken down into 7 days.
- You can do the week of workouts across any 7 days that works best for your schedule. For example, you could start day one on Monday or you could start it on Saturday.
- Look at the time commitment of each of the days and figure out the best way to fit it into your schedule.

For most people, starting day one on Monday makes the most sense. This is because day six is typically a more time-intensive workout, so doing that workout on a weekend usually works best for most schedules. Of course, feel free to adapt the schedule in a way that works best for you. For example, if you work weekends, having a weekday as your day six might be optimal.

## THE TIME-CRUNCHED PLAN (3 HOURS A WEEK)

This plan meets the government's exercise recommendations. It gives you a minimum but powerfully effective dose of walking with weight that'll kick-start your wellness journey and improve your health and performance. That makes it great for people just starting to exercise or who are short on time.

**Day 1:** Walk with weight for 30 minutes.
**Day 2:** Strength train for 30 minutes.
**Day 3:** Active recovery. Try to walk at least 7,000 steps.
**Day 4:** Walk with weight for 30 minutes.
**Day 5:** Strength train for 30 minutes.
**Day 6:** Walk with weight for 60 minutes.
**Day 7:** Active recovery. Try to walk at least 7,000 steps.

Repeat for up to 8 weeks.

**Note one:** Walk at a pace that feels challenging. If you can't do two separate 30-minute walks—day 1 and day 4—you can combine those days and do one 60-minute walk on either day 1 or 4. On the days you don't exercise, try to get 7,000 steps.

**Note two:** If you need to take a separate short walk to reach 7,000 steps on your rest days, feel free to throw on a lighter pack than the one you used for your walking-with-weight sessions. For example, if you used a 25-pound pack on days 1, 4, and 6, you could use a 15-pound pack. You don't have to do this, but feel free to if you want an added challenge.

**Note three:** Over the 8 weeks, try to improve. Increase your walking speed or the weight in your pack, or try to add weight to your strength-training exercises.

## THE MODERATELY BUSY PLAN (4.5 HOURS A WEEK)

This plan doubles the government's exercise recommendations. It's ideal for those who want to optimize their health and longevity in the least time possible.

**Day 1:** Walk with weight for 45 minutes.
**Day 2:** Strength train for 45 minutes.
**Day 3:** Active recovery. Try to walk at least 10,000 steps.
**Day 4:** Walk with weight for 45 minutes.
**Day 5:** Strength train for 45 minutes.
**Day 6:** Walk with weight for 90 minutes.
**Day 7:** Active recovery. Try to walk at least 10,000 steps.

Repeat for up to 8 weeks.

**Note one:** Walk at a pace that feels challenging. If you can't do two separate 45-minute walks—day 1 and day 4—you can combine those days and do one 90-minute walk on either day 1 or 4. On the days you don't exercise, try to get 10,000 steps.

**Note two:** If you need to take a separate short walk to reach 10,000 steps on your rest days, feel free to throw on a lighter pack than the one you used for your walking-with-weight sessions. For example, if you used a 30-pound pack on days 1, 4, and 6, you could use a 15- or 20-pound pack. You don't have to do this, but feel free to.

**Note three:** Over the 8 weeks, try to improve. Increase your walking speed or the weight in your pack, or try to add weight to your strength-training exercises.

## THE GO-GETTER PLAN (7 HOURS A WEEK)

This plan is geared toward someone who wants to really push their fitness. It's ideal if you're prepping for a fitness event, long backpacking trip, or just want to stay really fit. Don't jump into this plan if you're just starting to walk with weight. If you're just starting, begin with the 3-hour plan and work your way up.

**Day 1:** Walk with weight for 60 minutes.
**Day 2:** Strength train for 60 minutes.
**Day 3:** Active recovery. Try to walk at least 10,000 steps.
**Day 4:** Walk with weight for 60 minutes.
**Day 5:** Strength train for 60 minutes.
**Day 6:** Walk with weight for 120 minutes.
**Day 7:** 60 minutes of relaxed, non-impactful cardio, like swimming, cycling, or a stair step machine.

Repeat for up to 8 weeks.

**Note one:** Use an adequate weight, and walk at a pace that feels challenging.

**Note two:** If you need to take a separate short walk to reach 10,000 steps on your rest days, feel free to throw on a lighter pack than the one you used for your walking-with-weight sessions. For example, if you used a 30-pound pack on days 1, 4, and 6, you could use a 15- or 20-pound pack. You don't have to do this, but feel free to.

**Note three:** Over the 8 weeks, try to improve. Increase your walking speed or the weight in your pack, or try to add weight to your strength-training exercises.

## SAMPLE STRENGTH WORKOUTS

To access videos of the workouts and exercises described in the plans below, scan the following QR code:

### 30 minutes for the time-crunched plan

**Note:** This workout is quick and requires no gym equipment. You can use your weighted pack as a weight.

- **Two Percent Warmup** (see page 110)
- **Reverse Lunges with your weighted pack on:** 2 sets of 10 to 20 reps
- **Push-ups:** 2 sets of as many reps as you can do, stopping 3 reps short of failure—for example, if you could do 10 push-ups, you'd stop at 7
- **Hamstring Holds:** 2 sets of 10 reps
- **Weighted Pack Rows:** 2 sets of 10 to 20 reps
- **Plank:** 2 sets of 30- to 60-second holds

## 45 minutes for the moderately busy plan

**Note:** This workout requires equipment. If you'd rather use your pack as a weight, I've noted swaps below.

- **Two Percent Warmup** (see page 110)
- **Jumping Rope:** 3 minutes
- **Reverse Lunge with Dumbbells:** 3 sets of 10
- **Incline Dumbbell Bench Press:** 3 sets of 10
- **Hamstring Walkout:** 3 sets of 10
- **Dumbbell Row:** 3 sets of 10
- **Bird Dog:** 3 sets of 10

Swaps if you don't have weights: Do Reverse Lunges while wearing your pack instead of the Reverse Lunge with Dumbells; do push-ups with your pack on instead of the Dumbbell Bench Press; do rows with your pack instead of Dumbbell Rows.

## 60 minutes for the go-getter plan

**Note:** This plan has two separate workouts and requires equipment.

### Workout One

- **Two Percent Warmup** (see page 110)
- **Jumping Rope:** 3 minutes
- **Rear Foot Elevated Split Squat:** 3 sets of 10
- **Pull-up:** 3 sets of as many reps as possible, stopping 1 or 2 reps short of failure (if you can't do pull-ups, do Dumbbell Rows)
- **Floor Press:** 3 sets of 10
- **Hamstring Walkout:** 3 sets of 10
- **Dumbbell Pullover:** 3 sets of 10

- **Bird Dog:** 3 sets of 10
- **Farmer's Carry:** 3 sets of 100 steps

**Workout Two**

- **Two Percent Warmup** (see page 110)
- **Jumping Rope:** 3 minutes
- **Goblet Squat:** 3 sets of 10
- **Dumbbell Row:** 3 sets of 10
- **Single Arm Overhead Press:** 3 sets of 10
- **Kettlebell Swing:** 3 sets of 10
- **Dumbbell Pullover:** 3 sets of 10
- **Hanging Leg Raise:** 3 sets of as many reps as possible
- **Suitcase Carry:** 3 sets of 100 steps

# EPILOGUE

I wrote this book to make the case that the most powerful, underutilized, and fundamentally human form of exercise is simple: walking with weight.

I'm writing this epilogue after just finishing an 850-mile hike across one of the most remote, rugged landscapes in America—the Hayduke Trail. It's a route that snakes through the canyons and deserts of Utah and Arizona—summitting 11,000-foot mountains, exploring high and endless plateaus, and winding deep into labyrinth-like slot canyons. I had a pack on my back every single mile. Everything I needed to survive was in that pack.

The journey lasted roughly 45 days. There were blisters and blood, heat and hail, sunstroke and sagebrush, brutal climbs, and perspective-altering views. There were mornings I woke up freezing and nights coyotes crept into my campsite.

Through it all, I walked with weight. The hike expanded and solidified the words in this book.

A person can learn a lot by putting some weight on their back and one foot in front of the other for 850 miles. I learned to care for my feet and eat like it was a full-time job—a necessity to fuel all that walking with weight. I learned that my body is far more resilient than I thought, as is my mind. I learned to problem-solve issues in the moment with duct tape, grit, map and compass, and whatever ingenuity I could muster. I learned to read raw desert landscapes like a book and to appreciate run-down gas stations in the middle of nowhere as a form of metaphorical and literal salvation.

But more than that, I experienced that the human body is built to walk with weight. Ideally outside in beautiful places.

And that also showed me what the human body is *not* built for—the fluorescently lit, four-walled, pixelated chaos of modern life. We're not meant to be indoors in chairs, behind screens, and on couches all day. Those modern comforts are nice in the short term but, when overused, can hurt us in the long run. Instead, we're built to move under load, to persist, to roam and carry in the natural world and return stronger.

During my hike, I became leaner, stronger, and more resilient. I began weighing 182 pounds and ended at 167 pounds of solid muscle. Toward the end of the hike, I was walking nearly 40 miles a day for multiple days in a row. But those are just the measurable, ephemeral changes.

The real transformation was internal. Somewhere along the trip, I stopped hearing the usual mental chatter—the emails, the headlines, the bullshit—and started hearing myself again. I thought about the people I love, the work I care about, the person I want to be. The noise fell away, and what remained was clarity of body, mind, and spirit.

The elegant combination of mass on my back and momentum at my feet across a spectacular and unforgiving landscape did that.

For me, walking with weight isn't some new wellness trend. It's what humans were born to do. It's scalable, forgiving, meditative, and powerful. It's a return to being human.

For me, hiking the Hayduke Trail was proof: a stress test of everything in this book. If this book is the theory, the Hayduke Trail was the lab.

Walking with weight is about reconnecting—with your body, your mind, and the ancient rhythms that have shaped humanity—and becoming a better person in the process.

And you don't need to walk 850 miles through a sweltering, waterless desert to find that. You just need to put on a pack and walk out the door. Ideally soon.

*In the end, I believe we don't need more comfort or hacks. We need* more acts like walking with weight. We need more effort. More presence. More friction. More long miles under load. Because what's on the other side of that effort isn't just fitness. It's strength, clarity, and truth.

I hope this book gave you something useful—now please use it.

Lace up your shoes. Grab your pack. Add some weight. And start walking.

# ACKNOWLEDGMENTS

Thanks to Leah, my mom, Stockton, and Conway for walking with me and helping me navigate life.

Thanks to Jan Baumer and Steve Troha, my literary mother and father. I couldn't write books without you two!

Thanks to Diana Baroni and Emma Effinger for guiding this book.

Thanks to Matthew Benjamin, who expertly edited the weighted-walking section of *The Comfort Crisis* and helped the act gain popularity.

Thanks to Doug Kechijian, Trevor Kashey, and Kelly Starrett for their wisdom.

Thanks to everyone who reads this book and goes for a walk, especially while wearing a weighted backpack or vest.

# REFERENCES


### Chapter 1: Born to Carry

Bramble, D., & Lieberman, D. (2004). Endurance running and the evolution of *Homo*. *Nature, 432*, 345–352. https://doi.org/10.1038/nature03052

Gibbons, A. (2022). Human ancestors were walking upright 7 million years ago, ancient limb bone suggests. *Science*. Retrieved June 9, 2025, from https://www.science.org/content/article/human-ancestors-were-walking-upright-7-million-years-ago-ancient-limb-bone-suggests

Lieberman, D. E. (2014). *The story of the human body: Evolution, health, and disease*. New York: Knopf Doubleday.

McGee, W. J. (1898). The Seri Indians (Seventeenth Annual Report of the Bureau of American Ethnology to the Secretary of the Smithsonian Institution, 1895–96, pp. 1–344). Government Printing Office. Retrieved June 9, 2025, from https://www.gutenberg.org/files/49403/49403-h/49403-h.htm

Semaw, S., Rogers, M. J., Quade, J., Renne, P. R., Butler, R. F., Domínguez-Rodrigo, M., . . . Simpson, S. W. (2003). 2.6-million-year-old stone tools and associated bones from OGS-6 and OGS-7, Gona, Afar, Ethiopia. *Journal of Human Evolution, 45*(2), 169–177. https://doi.org/10.1016/S0047-2484(03)00093-9

Wiens, J. J. (2023). How many species are there on Earth? Progress and problems. *PLoS Biology, 21*(11), e3002388. https://doi.org/10.1371/journal.pbio.3002388

### Chapter 2: From Carrying to Walking with Weight in Packs

Ambrose, S. E. (1994). *D-Day: June 6, 1944: The climactic battle of World War II*. New York: Simon & Schuster.

Berecz, B., Cyrille, M., Casselbrant, U., Oleksak, S., & Norholt, H. (2020). Carrying human infants—An evolutionary heritage. *Infant Behavior and Development, 60*, 101460. doi:10.1016/j.infbeh.2020.101460

Easter, M. (2021). *The comfort crisis: Embrace discomfort to reclaim your wild, happy, healthy self.* New York: Rodale Books.

Knapik, J. J., Reynolds, K. L., & Harman, E. (2004). Soldier load carriage: Historical, physiological, biomechanical, and medical aspects. *Military Medicine, 169*(1), 45–56. https://doi.org/10.7205/milmed.169.1.45

Langley, M., & Suddendorf, T. (2020). Mobile containers are a keystone human innovation. *Evolutionary Anthropology, 29*(4), 195–208. https://doi.org/10.1002/evan.21857

Marshall, S. L. A. (1950). *The soldier's load and the mobility of a nation.* Washington, DC: Combat Forces Press.

Orr, R. M. (2010). The history of the soldier's load. *Australian Army Journal, 7*(2), 67–88. Retrieved from Australian Army Research Centre website.

Wang, W. J., & Crompton, R. H. (2004). The role of load-carrying in the evolution of modern body proportions. *Journal of Anatomy, 204*(5), 417–430. https://doi.org/10.1111/j.0021-8782.2004.00295.x pmc.ncbi.nlm.nih.gov+8pmc.ncbi.nlm.nih.gov+8researchgate.net+8

**Chapter 3: Lifespan and Healthspan**

Ainsworth, B. E., Haskell, W. L., Herrmann, S. D., Meckes, N., Bassett, D. R. Jr., Tudor-Locke, C., . . . Leon, A. S. (2011). 2011 compendium of physical activities: A second update of codes and MET values. *Medicine & Science in Sports & Exercise, 43*(8), 1575–1581. https://doi.org/10.1249/MSS.0b013e31821ece12

Coker, M. S., Ladd, K., Murphy, C. J., Ruby, B. C., Shriver, T. C., Schoeller, D. A., . . . Coker, R. H. (2021). Alaska backcountry expeditionary hunting promotes rapid improvements in metabolic biomarkers in healthy males and females. *Physiological Reports, 9*(1), e14682. https://doi.org/10.14814/phy2.14682

Global Burden of Disease 2019 collaborators. (2020). Global, regional, and national burden of low back pain and disability, 1990–2019: A systematic analysis for the Global Burden of Disease Study 2019. *The Lancet Rheumatology, 2*(5), e291–e301.

Hillman, C. H., Buck, S. M., Themanson, J. R., Pontifex, M. B., & Castelli, D. M. (2009). The effect of acute treadmill walking on cognitive control and academic achievement in preadolescent children. *Neuroscience, 159*(3), 1044–1054. https://doi.org/10.1016/j.neuroscience.2009.01.057

Holt-Lunstad, J., Smith, T. B., & Layton, J. B. (2010). Social relationships and mortality risk: A meta-analytic review. *PLOS Medicine, 7*(7), e1000316. https://doi.org/10.1371/journal.pmed.1000316

Hunter, M. R., Gillespie, B. W., & Chen, S. Y.-P. (2019). Urban nature experiences reduce stress in the context of daily life based on salivary biomarkers. *Frontiers in Psychology, 10* (722). https://doi.org/10.3389/fpsyg.2019.00722

Jessup, J. V., Horne, C., Vishen, R. K., & Wheeler, D. (2003). The effects of weighted vest walking and strength-training exercises on bone mineral density (BMD), balance, strength, and self-efficacy in older women. *Biological Research for Nursing, 4*(3), 171–180. https://doi.org/10.1177/1099800402239628

Klepeis, N. E., Nelson, W. C., Ott, W. R., Robinson, J. P., Tsang, A. M., Switzer, P., . . . Engelmann, W. H. (2001). The National Human Activity Pattern Survey (NHAPS): A resource for assessing exposure to environmental pollutants. Lawrence Berkeley National Laboratory. Retrieved June 9, 2025, from https://www.osti.gov/servlets/purl/785296

Knapik, J. J., Farina, E. K., Ramirez, C. B., Pasiakos, S. M., McClung, J. P., & Lieberman, H. R. (2019). Medical encounters during the United States Army Special Forces Assessment and Selection course. *Military Medicine.* Advance online publication. https://doi.org/10.1093/milmed/usz056

Knapik, J. J., Reynolds, K. L., & Harman, E. (2004). Soldier load carriage: Historical, physiological, biomechanical, and medical aspects. *Military Medicine, 169*(1), 45–56. doi:10.7205/milmed.169.1.45. PMID: 14964502

Lieben, M. (2017). Over nearly 80 years, Harvard study has been showing how to live a healthy and happy life. *Harvard Gazette.* Retrieved June 9, 2025, from https://news.harvard.edu/gazette/story/2017/04/over-nearly-80-years-harvard-study-has-been-showing-how-to-live-a-healthy-and-happy-life/

Looney, D. P., Lavoie, E. M., Notley, S. R., Holden, L. D., Arcidiacono, D. M., Potter, A. W., . . . Friedl, K. E. (2024). Metabolic costs of walking with weighted vests. *Medicine & Science in Sports & Medicine,. 56*(6), 1177–1185. doi:10.1249/MSS.0000000000003400

lululemon athletica inc. (2024). *2024 Global Wellbeing Report.* Retrieved June 9, 2025, from https://corporate.lululemon.com/~/media/Files/L/Lululemon/our-impact/lululemon-2024-global-wellbeing-report.pdf

Momma, H., Kawakami, R., Honda, T., & Sawada, S. S. (2022). Muscle-strengthening activities are associated with lower risk and mortality in major non-communicable diseases: A systematic review and meta-analysis of cohort studies. *British Journal of Sports Medicine, 56*(13), 755–764. https://doi.org/10.1136/bjsports-2021-104479

Mündermann, A., Nigg, B. M., Stefanyshyn, D. J., & Humble, R. N. (2005). Relationship between ground reaction force variables and peak knee compressive forces calculated using a mathematical model. *Clinical Biomechanics, 20*(5), 475–482.

Nguyen, T. H., Randolph, D. C., Talmage, J., Succop, P., & Travis, R. (2011). Long-term outcomes of lumbar fusion among workers' compensation subjects: A historical cohort study. *Spine, 36*(4), 320–331. https://doi.org/10.1097/BRS.0b013e3181ccc220

Orr, R. M., Pope, R. R., Johnston, V., & Coyle, J. (2010). Load carriage: Minimising soldier injuries through physical conditioning—A narrative review. *Journal of Military and Veterans' Health, 18*(3), 31–38. Retrieved from https://jmvh.org/article/load-carriage-minimising-soldier-injuries-through-physical-conditioning-a-narrative-review/

Ortega, F. B., Silventoinen, K., Tynelius, P., & Rasmussen, F. (2012). Muscular strength in male adolescents and premature death: Cohort study of one million participants. *British Medical Journal, 345*, e7279. https://doi.org/10.1136/bmj.e7279

Schoenfeld, B. J., Caramanica, L., Peterson, M. D., Contreras, B., Grgic, J., & Dankel, S. J. (2018). Muscular strength as a predictor of all-cause mortality in apparently healthy adults: A systematic review and meta-analysis. *Archives of Physical Medicine and Rehabilitation, 99*(11), 2299–2309. https://doi.org/10.1016/j.apmr.2018.04.006

Shcherbina, A., Mattsson, C. M., Waggott, D., Salisbury, H., Christle, J. W., Hastie, T., . . . Ashley, E. A. (2017). Accuracy in wrist-worn, sensor-based measurements of heart rate and energy expenditure in a diverse cohort. *Journal of Personalized Medicine, 7*(2), 3. https://doi.org/10.3390/jpm7020003

University of Pittsburgh, Research Center for Injury Prevention and Human Performance. (2010). Baseline injury surveillance and physical performance analysis in the 101st Airborne Division [Unpublished internal report, Blanchfield Army Community Hospital]. University of Pittsburgh.

U.S. Department of Health and Human Services. (2018). *Physical activity guidelines for Americans* (2nd ed.). Retrieved June 9, 2025, from https://health.gov/paguidelines/second-edition/pdf/Physical_Activity_Guidelines_2nd_edition.pdf

van Gent, R. N., Siem, D., van Middelkoop, M., van Os, A. G., Bierma-Zeinstra, S. M., & Koes, B. W. (2007). Incidence and determinants of lower extremity running injuries in long-distance runners: A systematic review. *British Journal of Sports Medicine, 41*(8), 469–480.

van Tulder, M., Becker, A., Bekkering, T., Breen, A., del Real, M. T. G., Hutchinson, A., . . . Kostova, D. (2006). European guidelines for the management of acute low back pain in primary care. *European Spine Journal, 15*(Suppl 2), S192–S300.

Wermers, R. A. (2018). Bone density in women: Women's wellness. Mayo Clinic News Network. Retrieved June 9, 2025, from https://newsnetwork.mayoclinic.org/discussion/womens-wellness-bone-density-in-women/

Yang, L., Zhang, X., Yuan, X., Xie, C., & Luo, H. (2023). Exercise interventions for patients with chronic low back pain: A systematic review of twenty exercise types and their effects on pain and physical function. *Frontiers in Public Health, 11*. https://doi.org/10.3389/fpubh.2023.1155225

**Chapter 4: Be SUPERMEDIUM**

Afshin, A., Forouzanfar, M. H., Reitsma, M. B., Sur, P., Estep, K., Lee, A., . . . GBD 2015 Obesity Collaborators. (2017). Health effects of overweight and obesity in 195 countries over 25 years. *New England Journal of Medicine, 377*(1), 13–27. https://doi.org/10.1056/NEJMoa1614362

Barrett-Connor, E., et al. (2005). BMI and all-cause mortality among 49,165 Canadian women aged 40–59. *Journal of Clinical Epidemiology, 58*(11), 1111–1116.

Dai, H., Alsalhe, T. A., Chalghaf, N., Riccò, M., Bragazzi, N. L., . . . Wu, J. (2020). The global burden of disease attributable to high body mass index in 195 countries and territories, 1990–2017: An analysis of the Global Burden of Disease Study. *PLOS Medicine, 17*(7), e1003198. https://doi.org/10.1371/journal.pmed.1003198

Felson, D. T., Zhang, Y., Hannan, M. T., Naimark, A., Weissman, B. N., Aliabadi, P., & Levy, D. (1992). Weight loss reduces the risk for symptomatic knee osteoarthritis in women: The Framingham Study. *Annals of Internal Medicine, 116*(7), 535–539. https://doi.org/10.7326/0003-4819-116-7-535 pubmed.ncbi.nlm.nih.gov

Iliodromiti, S., Celis-Morales, C. A., Lyall, D. M., Anderson, J., Gray, S. R., Mackay, D. F., . . . Sattar, N. (2018). The impact of confounding on the associations of different adiposity measures with the incidence of cardiovascular disease: A cohort study of 296,535 adults of white European descent. *European Heart Journal, 39*(17), 1514–1520. https://doi.org/10.1093/eurheartj/ehy057

Keller, K., & Engelhardt, M. (2014). Strength and muscle mass loss with aging process. Age and strength loss. *Muscles, Ligaments and Tendons Journal, 3*(4), 346–350. PMID: 24596700; PMCID: PMC3940510.

Larsson, S. C., & Burgess, S. (2021). Causal role of high body mass index in multiple chronic diseases: A systematic review and meta-analysis of Mendelian randomization studies. *BMC Medicine, 19*(1), 320. https://doi.org/10.1186/s12916-021-02188-x

Lauby-Secretan, B., Scoccianti, C., Loomis, D., Grosse, Y., Bianchini, F., & Straif, K., on behalf of the IARC Handbook Working Group. (2016). Body fatness and cancer—Viewpoint of the IARC Working Group. *New England Journal of Medicine, 375*(8), 794–798. https://doi.org/10.1056/NEJMsr1606602

Manson, J. E., Greenland, P., LaCroix, A. Z., Stefanick, M. L., Mouton, C. P., Oberman, A., . . . Siscovick, D. S. (2002). Walking compared with vigorous exercise for the prevention of cardiovascular events in women. *New England Journal of Medicine, 347*(10), 716–725. https://doi.org/10.1056/NEJMoa020245

Nishiguchi, S., Yamada, M., Michikawa, T., Koyama, T., Ogawa, E., Taniguchi, Y., . . . Suzuki, T. (2016). Effect of exercise and weight loss on physical function in obese older adults: A randomized controlled trial. *BMC Geriatrics, 16*, 69. https://doi.org/10.1186/s12877-016-0274-z

Panchal, S., et al. (2019). Low lean mass and mortality risk: A dose-response meta-analysis. *Journal of Cachexia, Sarcopenia and Muscle, 10*(6), 1070–1090. https://doi.org/10.1002/jcsm.12502

Prado, C. M., Baracos, V. E., McCargar, L. J., Mourtzakis, M., Mulder, K. E., Reiman, T., . . . Sawyer, M. B. (2007). Body composition as an independent determinant of 5-fluorouracil–based chemotherapy toxicity: A prospective cohort study. *Clinical Cancer Research, 13*(11), 3264–3268. https://doi.org/10.1158/1078-0432.CCR-06-3067

Rizzo, N. (2022). Fitness industry statistics 2021–2028 [market research]. RunRepeat. Retrieved June 9, 2025, from https://runrepeat.com/fitness-industry

Vasudevan, A., & Ford, E. (2022). Motivational factors and barriers towards initiating and maintaining strength training in women: A systematic review and meta-synthesis. *Prevention Science, 23*(4), 674–695. https://doi.org/10.1007/s11121-021-01328-2

**Chapter 5: How to Start**

Helton, G. L., Cameron, K. L., Zifchock, R. A., Miller, E., Neary, M. T., Goss, D. L., & Florkiewicz, E. (2019). Association between running shoe characteristics and lower extremity injuries in United States

Military Academy cadets. *American Journal of Sports Medicine, 47*(12), 2853–2862. https://doi.org/10.1177/0363546519870534

Knapik, J. J., Reynolds, K. L., & Harman, E. (2004). Soldier load carriage: Historical, physiological, biomechanical, and medical aspects. *Military Medicine, 169*(1), 45–56. https://doi.org/10.7205/MILMED.169.1.45

Li, S. W., Chan, O. H. T., Ng, T. Y., Kam, L. H., Ng, C. Y., Chung, W. C., & Chow, D. H. K. (2019). Effects of backpack and double pack loads on postural stability. *Ergonomics, 62*(4), 537–547. https://doi.org/10.1080/00140139.2018.1552764

**Chapter 6: Level Up**

Childers-Yost, S., & Rahman, T. (2017). The soldier's heavy load: How modern combat loads undermine military readiness and future force design. Center for a New American Security.

Cigarroa, I., Bravo-Leal, M., Petermann-Rocha, F., Parra-Soto, S., Concha-Cisternas, Y., Matus-Castillo, C., Vásquez-Gómez, J., Zapata-Lamana, R., Parra-Rizo, M. A., Álvarez, C., & Celis-Morales, C. (2023). Brisk walking pace is associated with better cardiometabolic health in adults: Findings from the Chilean national health survey 2016–2017. *International Journal of Environmental Research and Public Health, 20*(8), 5490. https://doi.org/10.3390/ijerph20085490

Hall, K. S., Shiroma, E. J., Carlson, S. A., Kerr, J., Reis, J. P., & Lee, I.-M. (2020). Brisk walking pace is associated with cardiometabolic health benefits independent of total steps per day: Cross-sectional analyses of 15,618 women. *PLOS One, 15*(7), e0235277. https://doi.org/10.1371/journal.pone.0235277

Imran, T. F., Orkaby, A., Chen, J., Selvaraj, S., Driver, J. A., Gaziano, J. M., & Djoussé, L. (2019). Walking pace is inversely associated with risk of death and cardiovascular disease: The Physicians' Health Study. *Atherosclerosis, 289*, 51–56. https://doi.org/10.1016/j.atherosclerosis.2019.08.001

Knapik, J. J., Reynolds, K. L., & Harman, E. (2004). Soldier load carriage: Historical, physiological, biomechanical, and medical aspects. *Military Medicine, 169*(1), 45–56. https://doi.org/10.7205/MILMED.169.1.45

Kujawa, M., Goerlitz, A., Rutherford, D., & Kernozek, T. W. (2020). Patellofemoral joint stress during running with added load in female runners. *International Journal of Sports Medicine, 41*(8), 556–563. https://doi.org/10.1055/a-1088-5467

Locke, E. A., & Latham, G. P. (2002). Building a practically useful theory of goal setting and task motivation: A 35-year odyssey.

*American Psychologist, 57*(9), 705–717. https://doi.org/10.1037/0003-066X.57.9.705

Marshall, S. L. A. (1950). *The soldier's load and the mobility of a nation.* Washington, DC: Combat Forces Press.

Myers, J., Prakash, M., Froelicher, V., Do, D., Partington, S., & Atwood, J. E. (2002). Exercise capacity and mortality among men referred for exercise testing. *New England Journal of Medicine, 346*(11), 793–801. https://doi.org/10.1056/NEJMoa011858

Orr, R. M., Pope, R. R., Johnston, V., & Coyle, J. (2010). Load carriage: Minimising soldier injuries through physical conditioning—A narrative review. *Journal of Military and Veterans' Health, 18*(3), 31–38. Retrieved from http://jmvh.org/article/load-carriage-minimising-soldier-injuries-through-physical-conditioning-a-narrative-review-2/

Rodríguez-Gutiérrez, E., Torres-Costoso, A., del Pozo Cruz, B., Núñez de Arenas-Arroyo, S., Pascual-Morena, C., Bizzozero-Peroni, B., & Martínez-Vizcaíno, V. (2024). Daily steps and all-cause mortality: An umbrella review and meta-analysis. *Preventive Medicine, 185*, 108047.

Sharpe, S. R., Holt, K. G., Saltzman, E., & Wagenaar, R. C. (2008). Effects of a hip belt on transverse plane trunk coordination and stability during load carriage. *Journal of Biomechanics, 41*(5), 968–976. doi:https://doi.org/10.1016/j.jbiomech.2007.12.018

Shih, Y.-L., Shih, C.-C., & Chen, J.-Y. (2020). The association between walking speed and risk of cardiovascular disease in middle-aged and elderly people in Taiwan, a community-based, cross-sectional study. *PLoS One 15*(7), e0235277. https://doi.org/10.1371/journal.pone.0235277

van Rijnsoever, F. J., Morens-Borgers, A., Beenackers, M. A., & Velema, E. N. (2021). Updating goal-setting theory in physical activity promotion: Specific yet challenging goals yield superior performance. *Health Psychology Review*. Advance online publication. https://doi.org/10.1080/17437199.2021.2023608

**Chapter 7: Support**

Berg, J. A., & Eisenhauer, C. (2024). Adult dehydration. In *StatPearls*. National Library of Medicine (U.S.). Retrieved June 9, 2025, from https://www.ncbi.nlm.nih.gov/books/NBK555956/

Birrell, S. A., & Hooper, R. H. (2007). Initial subjective load carriage injury data collected with interviews and questionnaires. *Military Medicine, 172*(3), 306–311. https://doi.org/10.7205/MILMED.172.3.306

Knapik, J. J., & Reynolds, K. L. (1997). Load carriage in military operations: A review of historical, physiological, biomechanical, and medical aspects (Report No. ADA330082). Defense Technical

Information Center. Retrieved from https://apps.dtic.mil/sti/citations/ADA330082

Knapik, J. J., Reynolds, K. L., Duplantis, K. L., & Jones, B. H. (1995). Friction blisters: Pathophysiology, prevention and treatment. *Sports Medicine, 20*(3), 136–147. https://doi.org/10.2165/00007256-199520030-00002

Reynolds, K. L., White, J. S., Knapik, J. J., Witt, C. E., & Amoroso, P. J. (1999). Injuries and risk factors in a 100-mile (161-km) infantry road march. *Preventive Medicine, 28*(2), 167–173. https://doi.org/10.1006/pmed.1998.0396

Stubbs, B., Koyanagi, A., & Thompson, T. (2016). The epidemiology of back pain and its relationship with depression, psychosis, anxiety, sleep disturbances, and stress sensitivity: Data from 43 low- and middle-income countries. *General Hospital Psychiatry, 43*, 63–70. https://doi.org/10.1016/j.genhosppsych.2016.09.008

U.S. Army Public Health Center. (2022). Foot marching and load-carriage injuries (CPHE-IP-Road-Marching-Injuries). Aberdeen Proving Ground, MD. Retrieved June 9, 2025, from https://phc.amedd.army.mil/PHC%20Resource%20Library/cphe-ip-road-marching-injuries.pdf

### Chapter 8: Packs, Vests, and Gear

Bobet, J., & Norman, R. W. (1984). Effects of load placement on back muscle activity in load carriage. *European Journal of Applied Physiology and Occupational Physiology, 53*(1), 71–75. https://doi.org/10.1007/BF00964693

Knapik, J. J., & Reynolds, K. L. (1997). Load carriage in military operations: A review of historical, physiological, biomechanical, and medical aspects (Report No. ADA330082). U.S. Army Research Institute of Environmental Medicine. https://apps.dtic.mil/sti/citations/ADA330082

Li, S. S. W., Chan, O. H. T., Ng, T. Y., Kam, L. H., Ng, C. Y., Chung, W. C., & Chow, D. H. K. (2019). Effects of backpack and double pack loads on postural stability. *Ergonomics, 62*(4), 537–547. https://doi.org/10.1080/00140139.2018.1552764

Maloiy, G. M. O., Heglund, N. C., Prager, L. M., Cavagna, G. A., & Taylor, C. R. (1986). Energetic cost of carrying loads: Have African women discovered an economic way? *Nature, 319*, 668–669. https://doi.org/10.1038/319668a0

### Chapter 9: Adopt a Two Percent Mindset

Berecz, B., Cyrille, M., Casselbrant, U., Oleksak, S., & Norholt, H. (2020). Carrying human infants—An evolutionary heritage. *Infant*

*Behavior and Development*, 60, 101460. https://doi.org/10.1016/j.infbeh.2020.101460

Clayton, R., Thomas, C., & Smothers, J. (2015). How to do walking meetings right. *Harvard Business Review*. Retrieved from https://hbr.org/2015/08/how-to-do-walking-meetings-right

Kling, H. E., Moore, K. J., Brannan, D., & Caban-Martinez, A. J. (2021). Walking meeting effects on productivity and mood among white-collar workers: Evidence from the Walking Meeting Pilot Study. *Journal of Occupational and Environmental Medicine, 63*(2), e75–e79. https://doi.org/10.1097/JOM.0000000000002098

Oppezzo, M., & Schwartz, D. L. (2014). Give your ideas some legs: The positive effect of walking on creative thinking. *Journal of Experimental Psychology: Learning, Memory, and Cognition, 40*(4), 1142–1152. https://doi.org/10.1037/a0036577

Paluch, A. E., Bajpai, S., Bassett, D. R. Jr., Carnethon, M. R., Ekelund, U., Evenson, K. R., . . . Fulton, J. E. (2022). Daily steps and all-cause mortality: A meta-analysis of 15 international cohorts. *The Lancet Public Health, 7*(3), e219–e228. https://doi.org/10.1016/S2468-2667(21)00302-9

**Chapter 10: Challenge Yourself**

Knapik, J. J., Reynolds, K. L., & Harman, E. (2004). Soldier load carriage: Historical, physiological, biomechanical, and medical aspects. *Military Medicine, 169*(1), 45–56. https://doi.org/10.7205/MILMED.169.1.45

Stout, S. E. (1921). Training soldiers for the Roman legion. *The Classical Journal, 16*(7), 423–431. https://doi.org/10.2307/3288082

Vegetius. (Translated by N. P. Milner). (1993). *Epitome of military science* (2nd ed.). Liverpool University Press. (Original work published ca. 4th century CE)

# INDEX

## X

# ABOUT THE AUTHOR

Michael Easter is the *New York Times* bestselling author of *The Comfort Crisis* and *Scarcity Brain*. He also writes *Two Percent with Michael Easter*, the top Substack newsletter on health and wellness. When he's not writing, he's in the desert outside Las Vegas, hiking with a pack on his back.